Drug Controversy in Sport

Drug Controversy in Sport

The Socio-Ethical and Medical Issues

Edited by R. S. Laura and S. W. White

Allen & Unwin

First published in 1991
Allen & Unwin Australia Pty Ltd
8 Napier Street, North Sydney, NSW 2059

National Library of Australia
Cataloguing-in-Publication entry:

The Drug controversy in sport.

  Includes index.
  ISBN 1 86373 072 9.

  1. Doping in sports. 2. Athletes—Drug use. I. Laura, R. S. (Ronald
  S.). II. White, S. W.

362.29088796

Set in 10/11pt Times by Adtype Graphics Pty Ltd, North Sydney
Printed by SRM Production Services, Malaysia

Foreword

There is nothing so inspiring as an athlete striving to achieve excellence, and nothing so disillusioning as an athlete who has used drugs to artificially enhance his or her performance.

The use of performance enhancing drugs makes a mockery of all the ideals that sport represents.

The use of drugs by sportsmen and women is not a recent problem, but it was catapulted into the international spotlight during the Seoul Olympics.

The scandals of the Seoul Olympic Games made us realise that action must be taken to protect the goal of personal excellence that is integral to competitive sport.

It is not only the ideals of sport that are being harmed by drugs, but also the athletes themselves. There are serious and potentially lethal health risks associated with the use of drugs. Our athletes put more than their careers at risk when they resort to their use.

The Drug Controversy in Sport is a stimulating book. Apart from raising public awareness of the problem of drug use in sport, it challenges society to reconsider some of its attitudes and assumptions. It points out that today's society covertly encourages the drug problem by social pressure, chauvinistic nationalism, media reporting and financial incentives for the winners.

We have to decide whether we truly believe that winning is not everything, and if so, act on our belief. Unless we make some decisions about sport's philosophical framework, we may find that laboratories will replace athletic endeavour in the sporting arena.

I commend the Hunter Academy of Sport on their valuable input into this informative insight into Drugs in Sport. The NSW Government and NIB Health Funds Ltd have jointly sponsored this book and royalties will be returned to the academy for further initiatives by its Education Committee.

The academy was the driving force behind Australia's first National Congress of Socio-Ethical and Medical Aspects of Drugs in Sport held in Newcastle in August, 1989.

The Congress Conclusions, which make up a vital part of this text, will result in a greater understanding of this serious problem and lay the groundwork for reform.

The Hon. R. B. Rowland Smith, MLC
NSW Minister for Sport, Recreation and Racing
April 1991

NIB Health Funds Ltd continue to take an interest in the health of the community, and the use of drugs in sport is no exception. We are alarmed at the continuing reports of disability and death associated with their use in young sportspeople in Australia, many of whom act as role models for rising youngsters with sporting talent. We are proud to support this superb outline of the problem, debated and documented in the Hunter Region for the benefit of Australian sport and the international sporting community.

C. Rogers
General Manager
NIB Health Funds Ltd
Newcastle
April 1991

Contents

Figures

Acknowledgements

The Hunter Academy of Sport would like to acknowledge the following supporters of the Congress:

Major Sponsors of the Congress
NIB Health Funds Ltd
New South Wales State Government

Corporate Sponsors
AeroPelican Air Services Pty Ltd
Australian Airlines
Eastern Airlines
Elizabeth's Restaurant and Convention Centre
Faculty of Medicine, University of Newcastle
Newcastle Beach International Motel
Newcastle City Council Tourist Information Centre
The Council of the City of Maitland
Top of Town Motel, Newcastle
Thrifty Rent-A-Car
University of Newcastle

Sponsors
Australian Sports Medicine Federation
Bayer Australia Ltd
Ciba-Geigy Australia Limited
Hunter Valley Wine Society
Sandoz Australia Pty Ltd
Schering Pty Ltd
(particularly for the Satellite Meeting)

The editors and chapter authors are grateful to the scientific referees who made important and constructive criticisms concerning the content of this book.

Finally, a special vote of thanks goes to the Hunter Postgraduate Medical Institute and in particular Mrs V (Lucy) Smith, the Coordinator of the Institute, and her team as the Conference Organisers. Mrs Ruth Barrett was a tower of strength in providing secretarial services to the Organising Committee. We would like also to express our appreciation to Ms Gai Gardner for her invaluable typing assistance in helping to prepare the manuscript. We are grateful to Mr Lloyd Waddy, Q.C. for his wonderful address at the Congress Dinner, and to Clinical Associate Professor Ted Hennessy of the University of Newcastle, through whom the Newcastle Club was made available for the Congress Dinner.

The Editors

Professor Ronald S. Laura BA, MDiv, MA, DPhil

Educated at the Universities of Harvard, St. John's College, Cambridge and Brasnose College, Oxford, Dr. Laura is currently Professor in Education at the University of Newcastle, was for three years Chairman of the Sports Medicine and Education Committee, Hunter Academy of Sport and is currently Director of the Human Performance Research Centre, N.S.W. A highly respected International bodybuilding judge for the IFBB, and a former World Champion in Powerlifting, he has over the past two decades conducted bodybuilding clinics in the U.S., U.K. and Australia on training and posing techniques. His recent book, *The Matrix Principle* with K. R. Dutton (Allen & Unwin) provides a revolutionary approach to weight training as an alternative to the use of performance-boosting drugs. He is well-known around the globe for his editorial contributions and regular features for bodybuilding and fitness magazines. Among the many bodybuilding magazines in which he publishes are: *Muscle & Fitness* (US), *Ultra-Fit* (UK), *Bodypower* (U.K.), and *Australian Fitness and Training*. The most recent of his twelve books, *The Matrix Principle* (co-authored with Prof. K. Dutton) and published by Allen & Unwin in 1991 introduces a revolutionary training technique for drug-free muscle development which has been acclaimed worldwide. Actively involved in the promotion of sports education in the public arena, he appears as a commentator on a number of television programs such as Wide World of Sport. He is also well-known for his role as master of ceremonies at major national and international sporting events, and he recently judged the World Bodybuilding Championships, held at the World Expo in Queensland.

Professor Saxon W White MB, BS, MD, FRACS

Saxon White is the Foundation Professor of Human Physiology at the new and innovative medical school at the University of Newcastle, NSW. He is a 4th generation Australian educated at the King's School, Parramatta, and at St Andrew's College and the University of Sydney, where at school and University he was a brilliant sportsman. He was NSW Schoolboys 440yd Champion and represented Combined Great Public Schools at cricket and rugby culminating in cricket and rugby blues at the University of Sydney. As an undergraduate he played rugby for NSW and toured twice overseas to South Africa and to the British Isles with the Australian Wallabies playing 29 games for Australia including seven test matches. He coached rugby at the University of New South Wales while reading for his higher doctorate in Medicine before continuing his postgraduate education in scientific medicine at the Universities of Göteborg (Sweden), California (San Diego, USA) and Oxford (UK). He has an international reputation as a medical scientist in the field of cardiorespiratory physiology and medicine and is the author of some 100 scientific papers and book chapters. In 1987 he was instrumental in creating the Hunter Academy of Sport, which he chairs. He plays cricket with I Zingari (Australia).

Participants

Mr James Barry
Board Member, Hunter Academy of Sport
Department of Sport, Recreation & Racing
Newcastle, N.S.W. 2300

Mr Alan Beard
Director of Education, Hunter Region
Newcastle, N.S.W. 2300

Professor Arnold Beckett
Medical Commission
International Olympic Committee
Wandsworth Plain
London, SW18 1EH, England

Senator John Black
Senate Standing Committee on Environment, Recreation
and the Arts
Canberra, A.C.T. 2601

Mr Ken Brown
Department of Sport, Recreation and Racing
North Sydney, N.S.W. 2060

Ms Adele Buchanan
Faculty of Medicine
University of Newcastle, N.S.W. 2308

Mr Terry Charlton
Board Member, Hunter Academy of Sport
PO Box 2136, Dangar, NSW 2309
Former Olympic basketball manager

Mr Ken Cole
Coach, Newcastle Falcons Basketball Team
Newcastle, NSW 2300

Mr Ken Clifford
Executive Officer
Hunter Academy of Sport
PO Box 2136, Dangar, NSW 2309

Mr Peter Collins, MP.
Minister for Health
Parliament House
Sydney, NSW 2000

Dr Brian Corrigan
Australian Sports Commission
Belconnen, ACT 2616

Dr David Cowan
Drug Control and Teaching Centre
London, SW3 6LX, England

Mr Alan Davis
Board Member, Hunter Academy of Sport
PO Box 2136, Dangar, NSW 2309

Professor Ken Donald
Professor of Pathology
John Hunter Hospital
New Lambton, NSW 2305
Former Australian Rugby International

Mr Leslie Eastcott
Board Member, Hunter Academy of Sport
PO Box 2136, Dangar, NSW 2309

Ms Dawn Fraser, MP.
Member for Balmain,
Balmain, NSW 2041
Former Olympic champion swimmer

Dr L Scott Frazier
Institute of Human Studies
Sherman Oaks, California 91403
United States of America

Dr Philip Furey
General Practitioner
11 Watt St, Newcastle, NSW 2300

Dr Robert Goldman
Amateur Athletic Union, Sports Medicine Committee
Chicago, Ill 60614
United States of America

Ms Marina Gielgud
Artistic Director
Australian Ballet Company
Melbourne, Vic 3000

Mr Steve Haynes
National Programme on Drugs in Sport
Belconnen, ACT 2616

Professor Vernon Howard
Harvard University
Cambridge, MA 02138
United States of America

Mr Craig Johnston
Soccer International
c/- NIB Health Funds Ltd
Newcastle, NSW 2300

Mr George Keegan, M.P.
Member for Newcastle
Newcastle, NSW 2300

Mr John Knipe
Board Member, Hunter Academy of Sport
PO Box 2136, Dangar, NSW 2309

Professor Ronald Laura
Professor of Education
University of Newcastle, NSW 2308
Former World Powerlifting Champion

Mrs Robyn Leggatt
Board Member, Hunter Academy of Sport
PO Box 2136, Dangar, NSW 2309
Former Australian Olympic women's hockey captain

Alderman John McNaughton
Lord Mayor of Newcastle
Newcastle, NSW 2300

Mr Norman May
International sports commentator
Potts Point, NSW 2011

Dr Tony Millar
Institute of Sports Medicine
Lewisham, NSW 2049

Mr Henry Meskausas
Maitland Council
Board Member, Hunter Academy of Sport
PO Box 2136, Dangar, NSW 2309

Dr P. G. Moore
Faculty of Medicine
University of Newcastle, NSW 2308

Mr Jack Newton
International golfer and commentator

Mr Hayden Opie
Faculty of Law
Melbourne University
Melbourne, Vic 3000

Mr Wayne Pearce
Rugby League International
Balmain Leagues Club
Balmain, NSW 2041

Dr Tony Quail
Faculty of Medicine
University of Newcastle, NSW 2308

Mr Mark Richards
Four times world surfing champion
Newcastle, NSW 2300

Mr Colin Rogers
General Manager
NIB Health Funds Ltd
Newcastle, NSW 2300

Professor David Russell
University of Otago
Dunedin, New Zealand

Dr John Sage
Board Member, Hunter Academy of Sport
PO Box 2136, Dangar, NSW 2039

Dr Brian Sando
President
Australian Sports Medicine Federation
Bruce, ACT 2617

Mr Bob Rowland Smith, M.P.
Minister for Sport, Recreation and Racing
Parliament House
Sydney, NSW 2000

Ms Helen Smith
Board Member, Hunter Academy of Sport
PO Box 2136, Dangar, NSW 2039

Mr George Souris, M.P.
Member for Upper Hunter
Muswellbrook, NSW 2333

Dr Dick Telford
Australian Institute of Sport
Belconnen, ACT 2616

Miss Elizabeth Toohey
Senior Artist
Australian Ballet Company
Melbourne, Vic 3000

Mr Tom van der Touw
Faculty of Medicine
University of Newcastle, NSW 2308

Mr Lloyd Waddy, Q.C.
180 Phillip Street
Sydney, NSW 2000

Mr Ivan Welsh, M.P.
Mayor
City of Lake Macquarie
Boolaroo, NSW 2284

Mr Alex Watson
Olympic Pentathlete
Halls Road
Galston, NSW 2159

Professor Saxon White
Professor of Human Physiology
University of Newcastle, NSW 2308
Former Australian Rugby International

Mr Dave Williams
Board Member, Hunter Academy of Sport
PO Box 2136, Dangar NSW 2309

Prolegomenon

The Hunter Region in Australia is the enormous Hunter River Valley and surrounding mountain margins and communities 160 kms north of Sydney. In 1988, the Hunter Academy of Sport was formed in response to the needs of the half million people of the Region. The remit was to coordinate the sporting service, education and research facilities of such cities as Newcastle, Lake Macquarie, Maitland, Singleton and Cessnock, and of the country areas around. This goal encompassed children, adults and the ageing, and was linked to the provision of better health. A comprehensive rural, industrial and university microcosm of Australia, the Hunter Region has a rich sporting and cultural history: for this reason both the Academy and Hunter community were depressed and confused by the drug-related events at the Seoul Olympic Games when an Australian pentathlete, Alex Watson, and overseas athletes such as Ben Johnson, fell from grace as an outcome of the drug testing weapons of modern chemistry.

At that time the Education Committee of the Academy, led by Professor Ronald Laura, recommended that the 1st Congress of the Academy should explore the issue of drugs in sport, and seek to understand not only the contemporary thinking and application of testing systems embraced by the International Olympic Committee, but to encompass the new understanding of physiology and genetics in our view of the athlete of the future, and how this should sit with a more informed International Olympic Committee and its modern policies.

To this end, on 22–25 August 1989, some 200 people made up of regional, national and international delegates, speakers and press, attended the 1st National Congress on Socio-Ethical and Medical Aspects of Drugs in Sport, held under the auspices of the Hunter Academy of Sport, and sponsored by the New South Wales Government's Department of Sport, Recreation and Racing, and by NIB Health Funds Limited. The Congress was held at Queen's Wharf, and at the David Maddison Building within the precincts of the Royal Newcastle Hospital in Newcastle.

This book highlights the important and unique contributions made at the Congress. It is an expression of the need for a sport-minded antipodean society to document the multifaceted and authentic views of politicians, philosophers, scientists, physicians, and athletes about a serious and hidden problem in its midst.

The goals of the Academy in promoting the Congress were:

• To provide an educational forum during which experts who deal with performance boosting aids (chiefly drugs) will interface with the general public, athletes, coaches, and the public administration.

• To establish the history of performance boosting aids, current practice and their potentiality in the future.

• To identify current policy with respect to the use of performance boosting aids at an international, national, state and Hunter Region level.

• To review the evidence for performance enhancement by such aids, incorporating elements of their pharmacology, their effects on human physiology and of side-effects.

• To discuss ethical and legal issues of doping in sport and the performing arts.

• To identify test procedures, their accuracy, where they are carried out, and their relevance to current and future policy.

• To document the main conclusions and recommendations of the forum in order to stimulate policy discussions at least within the Hunter Region, and in the State of New South Wales.

The main Congress was formulated as a mainstream program of speakers, who then with the audience formed small groups first to define the problems emerging, and on a second occasion to try and resolve the issues.

In addition, two public meetings were held at night, and these were attended on each occasion by a packed audience. The first public meeting was chaired by Mr Norman May, international Australian sports commentator, and was entitled 'The Drug Controversy in Sport: Should We Be Plugged In?' The second was in the form of an hypothetical entitled 'The Birth of Superman' and was moderated by Professor Ronald Laura. These brilliant evenings were recorded and published as manuscripts* complementary to this book by the Academy's major sponsor, NIB Health Funds Ltd. The discussion panel on each occasion was invited, and comprised prominent Australian and international athletes, coaches, administrators and civic leaders. This gave the athletes in particular a chance to express their views in public. For example, Alex Watson never denied he drank coffee at Seoul during the Pentathlon; but he left no doubt in the minds of the audience that our athletes were short of accurate guidelines and pre-competition advice from officials and above all, from coaches, when it came to implementing the rules and penalties emanating from contemporary IOC policy. From the debate between Alex and Brian Corrigan, and the comments from Arnold Beckett and David Cowan, the view emerged that IOC policy was predominantly protective and punitive and aimed at testing for drugs, the effects of which, e.g. in the case of caffeine, as true enhancers of performance are still highly controversial. The burgeoning efficiency and enormous cost of detection internationally *in the absence of a soundly based public expectation of the athlete's behaviour, suggested that the IOC tail was wagging the IOC dog.*

An unexpected revelation came from Elizabeth Toohey of the Australian Ballet, who revealed best the philosophical paradox of the contemporary high performing athlete. The extraordinary consistency of prowess and aesthetics demanded of dancers over weeks, months and years in the current Australian Ballet (demanded by themselves of themselves) left no place for drugs which may interfere with the *quality of the performance, and their physical appearance.* Miss Toohey also claimed the dancers were non-competitive; but she did say they competed 'against themselves', that there were such things as ballet Olympics, and in this competition there could be little margin for technical error. Then we all saw and heard Marina Gielgud, her 'coach', on video immediately after Miss Toohey's major address. There before us sat an artistic director of reputation and qualities of leadership guiding a company growing in international stature. If Elizabeth Toohey reflected the philosophy, morale and drive for perfection of the rest of the Company, we would support the notion of Toohey for the 100 metres at Barcelona, and Gielgud for the coach of the Women's Track and Field. This would be a drug-free team.

There was a Satellite meeting immediately following the main Congress on Saturday, 26 August 1989, targeted through the Hunter Postgraduate Medical Institute at regional medical practitioners, who for professional reasons could not attend during the week. The meeting illuminated one of the key interface areas for

the education of the public, for the management of athletes who
seek drugs or become ill from taking drugs, and which represents a
potential source of drugs. In 1991 the need for general practitioners to understand the drug problem in sport grows daily as
more and more reports come in from athletes indeed dying from
drug misadventure in Australian sport. A special mention must be
made of Dr Tony Millar and Dr Philip Furey, for their thoughtful
and professional contributions concerning ethics and management
to the medical profession, e.g. at the Royal Newcastle Hospital
Grand Rounds during the Congress and Satellite meetings. One
excellent outcome of the Congress has been the inclusion of a
special segment on drugs in sport in the fourth year of the undergraduate curriculum at the Medical School of the University of
Newcastle.

The main recommendation was presented by Arnold Beckett and
David Cowan on behalf of the Hunter Academy of Sport at the 2nd
Permanent World Congress of Drugs in Sport in Moscow, October
1989, and the Congress outcomes are now widely in the hands of
government and the public.

It is difficult to judge the extent to which the recommendations
will influence society, given the dynamics of IOC, Government,
Australian Sports Drug Agency and personal policy making, some
of which was already changing when the Congress was held. Nevertheless, it is the Academy's hope that publishing the content and
ebb and flow of debate at the Congress will bring a wider understanding of what continues to emerge as a *real* and growing human
problem, but one which still appears to be mainly hidden in the
recesses of the locker room. All the evidence, such as it is, suggests
the problem is becoming worse in Australia, and internationally.
We believe the unique cluster of politics, science and philosophy in
this book is at the same instant both contemporary, and timeless.

S. W. White, R. S. Laura
Hunter Academy of Sport
April 1991

* The Public Forum, chaired by Norman May, was entitled 'The Drug-Sport Connection: Should We Be Plugged in?'. The Hypothetical, moderated by Ron Laura,
was entitled 'The Birth of Superman'. The comprehensive Transcripts of these two
public meetings are available from the Executive Officer, The Hunter Academy of
Sport, PO Box 2136, Dangar, NSW, 2309, Australia. Cost to overseas readers is
$US20.00 plus return airmail postage. Cost to Australian readers is $A20.00.

1 The price athletes pay in pursuit of Olympic gold
Ronald Laura and Saxon White

Whether the Olympic Games will survive the onslaught of drug abuse which continues to taint them has come to constitute a major issue within the world of sport, making the future and social value of sport itself, uncertain.

During the 1988 Olympics in Seoul the public witnessed the expulsion and dishonour of some of the world's top athletes on charges of doping. The Bulgarian weight-lifting team felt constrained to pack up and return home after two of its medallists tested positive for the diuretic, furosemide. The public promptly learned that furosemide is used to flush water rapidly from the body, thus enabling an athlete to reduce those last few kilos of bodyweight which would otherwise prevent him/her from competing in a lower weight class. Australia's pentathlete, Alex Watson, was expelled from the Games—amidst controversy—after his urine test revealed an illegally high level of caffeine.

Given that caffeinated coffee is commonly drunk as a social beverage, we tend not to think of caffeine as a performance-boosting drug. However, those advertisements which extol that 'Coke or Pepsi feeling' serve to make the point that caffeine and its family of chemical relatives, the *xanthines,* are a source of potent stimulants to the central nervous system. Since caffeine can improve alertness and possibly endurance, stave off mental fatigue, and even steady a shaky hand, it is unsurprising that some athletes might be tempted to use caffeine as an ergogenic (an artificial aid reputed to enhance athletic performance). Given the wide range of socially acceptable beverages in which caffeine is found, and the different rates at which caffeine is metabolised by particular individuals, the level of caffeine prohibited by the International Olympic Committee may be ambiguous. The caffeine anomaly is just one of the many difficulties for the IOC in their admirable efforts to set objective and fair criteria for the detection of prohibited doping substances.

Following Watson's expulsion from the Games a second pentathlete, this time from Spain, was also expelled for alleged drug use. By the end of the first week of competition in Seoul the number of drug-related disqualifications had soared to ten, thus approximating the number of disqualifications for similar violations in the 1984 Games. The melodrama of disqualifications might have been forgotten or at least overshadowed by other great performances, were it not for the steroid controversy surrounding the legendary Ben Johnson of Canada, the third gold medallist to fail the drug tests at Seoul.

While all Olympic events have a certain appeal, there is something almost magical, if not sacred, about the 100 metre final. For many people the event typifies the spirit of the Olympic movement itself, providing for spectators of all sexes and nationalities a universally simple and basic form of competition with which they can all identify. It took Ben Johnson only 9.79 seconds to run the 100 metres and become the fastest man on earth, the hero of sporting heroes; it took only twelve or so hours to assay the urine samples which would expose Johnson as a cheat and stain his Olympic sporting future with disgrace.

The resounding condemnation of Johnson around the globe drew attention not only to the drug problem in sport but also to the philosophical framework of illusions which have come to define contemporary sport. The 'shock' and 'shame' attitude of sports administrators and the media reflected not so much the horror of Johnson's act of doping, as the horror of what sport has become. The traditional values of striving for excellence as a mark of personal achievement and self-discovery have been exchanged for the goal of winning at all costs, even the cost of personal integrity. The excellence is still there, it is to be admitted, but the battle being fought for excellence is now being directed by an army of chemists who wage a pharmaceutical war for supremacy among themselves. Will the Olympic Games of the 21st Century amount to little more than a pharmaceutical struggle; a race to prop up athletes with ever more effective drugs, and to devise other drugs to mask the drugs athletes have taken?

Ben Johnson's shame was symptomatic of a deeper malaise affecting all sport, but particularly Olympic sport, which pretends to set the example to which all amateur sport aspires. The problem is that Olympic sport has come to reflect in part our society's obsession with big business, and big business is what the Olympics has in part become. The television rights to the Olympic Games are now customarily marketed to the TV media barons of the world: they went, in 1988, to the highest bidder for $US500 million. It would be naive to pretend that the modern Olympic Games and the athletes who participate in them are unaffected by vested interests and the consumer mentality that inspires them. There is a persistent irony in the fact that athletes such as Ben Johnson are regarded by the IOC as amateur sports persons, though they have in fact amassed considerable fortunes by playing sport. Not unlike many other top amateur athletes around the world, Johnson's sporting success and his post-Olympic career— 1990–91 have been inextricably linked with his success in marketing, promoting, and advertising his skills in the form of a viable commercial product. That many sporting personalities employ a business agent to advance and manage their sporting careers bears witness to the extent to which sport and big business have become entangled.

Winning at all costs is not simply a matter of being willing *to do anything* to win just for the sake of winning. The issue has become far more complicated and perverse; it has become a matter of recognising that there is a *financial cost* in not winning. To put it another way: Ben Johnson not only made it his goal to become the fastest man on earth; he made it his *business* to become the fastest man on earth. His win was valued enough on the commercial market that despite having been stripped of his gold medal and publicly dishonoured, he was quickly offered lucrative contracts to play gridiron football for both Canadian and American teams. His return to competitive running in 1991 has been marked by appearance fees of up to $100 000, and *he* estimates his two-year disgrace cost him $25 million in lost contracts.

The history of doping in sport

One misconception about the role played by drugs in sport is that ergogenic aids appeared on the sports scene only in the early 1950s, due largely to the desire of competitive bodybuilders and weight-lifters for success in their respective sports. This may be a reasonably accurate picture of the introduction of anabolic steroids, but it belies the fact that doping has been a pervasive part of sport for more than two millennia,[1] and the commitment to performance-boosting aids can be traced even further. It is only recently that certain peoples have abandoned the practice of dining on the viscera of their slain enemies, in the hope of inheriting their strength and courage.[2] It has been reported that by the fourth century BC competitors in sport followed the lead of soldiers and of the earlier Roman gladiators in preparing themselves for their tasks by dining on hallucinogenic mushrooms, assorted psychoactive seeds and herbal stimulants.[3] Winning, as they used to say in the gladiator arena, is not everything—'it is the only thing'.

By the mid-1800s athletes used ergogenics such as alcohol, caffeine, sugar-nitroglycerine (a compound of sugar soaked in nitroglycerine, a derivative of which is also used medically to arrest cardiac pain by improving the ratio of blood supply to meet metabolism in the heart muscle), opium, and even ethyl ether, all with the aim of improving their physical capabilities. A late 19th century drink called the 'wine for athletes', otherwise known as *vin Mariani,* was a widely used mixture of coca leaf extract and wine. By the turn of the 20th century the stimulant strychnine was added to the list and commonly combined with brandy to make the heady cocktail alleged to have helped the American, Thomas Hicks, gain victory in the 1904 St. Louis marathon. The price Hicks paid for his win was high. He collapsed at the end of the race and was on the brink of death for a considerable period.[4]

By the mid-1950s stimulant drugs such as amphetamines and sympathomimetic amines were taken by athletes in the hope of improving endurance and increasing energy for those last-minute bursts of strength required for a competitive advantage. In 1958 it was reported by the American College of Sports Medicine that 35 per cent of 441 trainers, coaches, and assistants had either personally used amphetamines or at least knew how to use them.[5] A 1961 survey by the Italian Association of Football revealed that psychotonic drugs were being used by 17 per cent of their athletes and that a staggering 94 per cent of players from the A-league club used drugs of some kind to enhance sporting performance.[6]

The escalation of drug misuse within the world of sport reached a major crisis point in the 1960 Olympic Games in Rome when the Danish cyclist Knut Enemark Jensen died from the misuse of stimulants taken to enhance his performance. Jensen's death was not only unnecessary, but a consequence of being medically ill-advised. He was taking Ronical tablets in addition to amphetamines on the assumption that they would increase blood flow through his muscles.[7] The heat of the Rome Olympics, coupled with the drugs he had taken, proved to be a fatal combination.

In 1965, sporting organisations in France and Belgium, gravely concerned that the increasing use of drugs was not only undermining the moral integrity of sport but had come to constitute a potentially lethal health hazard, petitioned successfully to secure antidoping legislation for their countries.[8] Despite these early efforts to control and discourage drug usage, the death in 1967 from amphetamines of British cyclist Tommy Simpson during the Tour de France competition was a stern reminder that the eradication of drugs in sport would be no easy matter. It was in this context of consternation that the present International Olympic Committee Medical Commission was established. As Arnold Beckett described the Commission's role:

The first task of the IOC Medical Commission was to consider the philosophy of control and types of drugs to be classed as doping agents, and then to establish suitable methods for testing. It took a pragmatic approach, namely to protect the competitor but to allow medication so long as a clear line could be drawn between acceptable and nonacceptable drugs in sport. It was fully recognised that not all doctors and coaches considered the welfare of competitors under their care to be the first priority. Pressures to succeed at all costs were in evidence in top-class sport. If competitions in sport were to become competitions between pharmacologists and physicians, with competitors being used as guinea pigs and receiving potent drugs, then inevitably there would be more deaths in sport ... [9]

With the introduction of drug-testing for the first time at the Mexico Olympics and the Grenoble Winter Games in 1968, the desperation of athletes to find performance-boosting alternatives to the easily detectable amphetamine-based stimulants led to a much greater emphasis on anabolic steroids. Synthetic modifications of the male sex hormone, including testosterone and anabolic steroids, were heralded as chemical aids capable of producing massive gains in muscular development and strength. Developed in the 1930s, steroids were first used in the service of medicine, providing a legitimate form of treatment for hormonal disorders and the repair of damaged tissue, including skeletal muscles. Their first non-medical use may have been prompted by Nazi doctors who made them available to German troops, on the assumption that anabolic steroids would make them more aggressive and facilitate muscle recuperation, especially in respect of muscle injury.

Cognisant of the Nazis use of steroids as a kind of performance enhancer, Soviet sports doctors and officials encouraged the use of steroids amongst their athletes in the early 1950s, achieving a modest measure of improved performance for Soviet competitors. It was in 1956 that Dr John Ziegler discovered that the Russians were administering their athletes with performance-boosting drugs, including injections of straight testosterone.[10] It is reported that

the health of some of the young Soviet athletes receiving testosterone shots was so badly affected that they had to be catheterised in
order to urinate.

Ziegler returned to the US and worked prodigiously on the development of the more sophisticated form of anabolic steroids available today. Because of the health risks involved, he had hoped to
improve on the doping substances then in use by the Russians,
while at the same time providing American athletes with a more
efficient ergogenic agent. Ziegler soon came to realise that the
creation of steroids was tantamount to the creation of a monster
which would be difficult, if not impossible to control. Once the US
discovered the alleged competitive advantage gained by Soviet athletes from steroids, the chemical coldwar began and America athletes began taking steroids in quantities far beyond the
recommended doses.

As early as the 1964 Games anabolic steroids had become a part
of the performance-boosting program of Olympic athletes. Professor Manfred Donike, chief of the West German antidoping laboratory and a member of the IOC Medical Commission, recalls that at
the 1964 Tokyo Olympics there were reports of the toilets being
'littered with vials and syringes'.[11]

Testifying before a US Senate Committee in 1973, Harold
Connelly, four-time competitor and gold medalist in the hammer-
throw, commented:

> It was not unusual in 1968 to see athletes with their own medical
> kits, practically a doctor's, in which they would have syringes and all
> their various drugs ... I know any number of athletes on the 1968
> Olympic team who had so much scar tissue and so many puncture
> holes in their backsides that it was difficult to find a fresh spot to
> give them a new shot.[12]

By the time of the 1976 Montreal Olympics steroid usage among
Olympic athletes had become not only rampant, but blatant. When
observers noted that a number of women from the East German
swim team seemed possessed of several vaguely masculine features, including particularly deep voices, their coach unabashedly
replied, 'We have come here to swim, not sing.'[13] Having defected
to the West in 1977, the famous East German female sprinter,
Renate Neufeld', revealed that when she refused to take 'hormone
pills' she was threatened with reprisals and forced to undergo
psychotherapy.[14]

Although the IOC had begun testing for steroids at the 1976
Olympics, the statistics on offenders have not always accurately
reflected the true situation of doping violation. There is first of all
the problem that testing methods have what might be called an

almost inevitable 'built-in obsolescence'. Once the testing procedures for amphetamines were developed, thus ensuring a relatively easy detection of these substances in the urine, athletes simply substituted undetectable doping substances for the detectable ones. As soon as the IOC tests for steroids were developed, athletes began injecting testosterone, for example, a substance for which no test was available until 1981. For those unable to satisfy that winning hunger with steroids, *blood doping* provided another untestable option. It was at the Montreal Olympics in 1976 that Lasse Viren of Finland established his supremacy as one of the world's greatest long-distance runners—and, it was rumoured, as the crown prince of blood doping.[15]

Blood doping is a performance-boosting technique in which blood is taken from an athlete well in advance of a competition and preserved in a frozen, concentrated form. Just prior to the competition, the extra blood cells are injected back into the body, allegedly increasing the oxygen carrying capacity of the cells by as much as 20 per cent. Whether or not the rumours about Viren were true remains an unsolved mystery, but there is little doubt that Viren's success, and the belief on the part of his competitors that his success was due largely to blood doping, prompted many athletes to try the technique themselves. Since no foreign substances are involved, there is no easy way of proving that the technique has been used to gain an unfair advantage.

The second problem in relation to drug testing, is that athletes, knowing they are to be tested, are able to take steps to ensure that the tests will not return positive. It would seem that the use of doping substances is far more widespread than the disqualification for doping indicates. Dr Robert Voy, Chief Medical Officer for the US Olympic Committee, reported that in 1983–84 no-penalty testing revealed, for instance, that between 20 and 50 per cent of US athletes were doping.[16] These figures contrast markedly to the current rate of 2 to 3 per cent of athletes whose *formal* tests prove positive at competition time. Such a disparity would indicate that many athletes are managing to beat the tests, reputedly either by taking other drugs which mask the presence of prohibited drugs, or by cutting back on the prohibited performance-boosting drugs in time to clear their systems of detectable foreign substances.

The 1980 Moscow Games constituted another statistical aberration. Not one of the 2200 Olympic competitors tested positive for doping violations, whereas eleven out of 2061 athletes were disqualified at the previous Montreal Olympics in 1976, while eleven out of 1520 competitors proved positive for doping violations at the subsequent Olympics held in 1984 at Los Angeles.[17]

That, in the 1980s, Moscow alone was able to host a drug-free Olympics must be regarded as a truly remarkable, if not incredible, achievement.

As the tests for steroids became more rigorous, the search for increasingly effective and even less detectable performance-boosting agents has led to an escalation in the development of drugs which mimic as closely as possible those chemical substances associated with human performance which occur naturally within the body. The current trend includes synthetic and genetically engineered forms of human growth hormone (HGH) and human chorionic gonadotrophin (HCG). Children suffering from hormonal deficiencies associated with growth disorders have traditionally been treated with HGH. Using HGH to increase size and strength in adults, however, can produce a number of side-effects, such as diabetes, hepatitis and acromegaly, a disorder of the pituitary associated with enlarged hands and feet, thickened lips and tongue, and facial distortions including a jutting lower jaw.

HCG is a substance derived from the urine of pregnant women. It is supposed to facilitate muscular development by stimulating the natural production of testosterone within the male body. One peculiarity of HCG is that when the males who use it are drug-tested, their urine analysis reveals not only that they are taking drugs, but that *they are pregnant*. This persistent emphasis upon drugs in sport has finally given rise to the maxim, 'anabolic steroids, sprinkled with HGH and a little HCG, are the breakfast of champions'. The truth expressed gives a whole new and tragic sense of an older maxim, 'We are what we eat.'

The progressive reliance upon genetic engineering techniques, including recombinant DNA techniques, is ushering in a whole new era in the development of performance-boosting aids. In addition to the manufacture of growth hormone, genetic engineering may soon be commonly used to make 'endorphins' and to clone specific cells whose proliferation could enhance performance. The IOC is likely in the future to face a new set of doping problems whose resolution could be far more difficult than the current drug problem.

Winning at all costs

In a much publicised interview big Steve Courson (6'1", 140 kg), who played 'offensive guard' for the Tampa Bay Buccaneers in Florida, is quoted as saying: 'The strongest people—the strongest athletes—in the world are all using steroids. They're being used not only in the strength field, but also in track and field and swimming. So you've got to be on drugs if you want to survive.'[18] In September 1987 at the World Track and Field Championships in Rome, Carl Lewis, multi-gold medal winner at the 1984 and 1988 Olympic Games, is quoted as saying 'There are gold medallists at this meet who are on drugs. Everybody knows it. It's obvious.'[19] It was in the same year that three Polish athletes scheduled to compete in the World Powerlifting Championships in Fredrikstad, Norway, were caught with some 9000 doses of anabolic steroids. To add to the scandal, an eventual class winner of the same meet who hailed from Belgium was arrested by Norwegian officials for being in possession of $US34 000 worth of steroids and testosterone.[20] Nor is steroid use limited to bodybuilders and strength athletes, including their field and track brethren. In February 1988 one of Poland's most celebrated hockey players was banned from the Calgary Winter Olympics on the basis of positive tests for anabolic steroids.[21]

Nor are male athletes alone in their use of steroids to boost performance, as is made clear by Professor Wildor Hollmann, President of the World Federation of Sport Medicine in Cologne, who was reported as saying, 'I believe that today there are few women's world records in running, high jump, broad jump, shot put, discus and possibly javelin that have come about without the help of anabolic steroids.'[22]

The number of top-level athletes caught in possession of anabolic steroids has in recent years also soared, despite the introduction of legal penalties.

The presumption in favour of doping is not an anomaly peculiar to US and European athletes. Within smaller countries such as Australia it is not unusual for gym owners to be bombarded with literature in which steroids are hailed as the panacea to Australian sporting ills. In one booklet now widely circulated to gyms in Australia the anonymous authors write:

Australia has always had good athletes and it is often said of Australians by Americans and Europeans that they (the other countries) are lucky that we (Australia) do not know how to use steroids ... So before anyone criticises our efforts to supply the best up to date information and to encourage, yes we encourage, the real athletes to take the step confidently ... check with the rest of the world and its class athletes before making biased decisions which will suppress Australia's impact for another ten years ...

The black market for doping in sport

On 4 October, 1987 Sydney's *Sun-Herald* newspaper published an expose of a massive gymnasium black market in anabolic steroids thriving within Australia. Black-market steroids are big business too, and even some top-class athletes have succumbed to the temptation to become pushers of the drug. It was in 1987 that David Jenkins, a British Olympic silver medallist, pleaded guilty in San Diego to the charges of his involvement in a $US140 million-a-year black market in steroids.[24] The possible connection between the sales outlets for steroids and hard drugs is a concern to many. The main concern is that the criminal element selling hard drugs has now moved into the lucrative black market in steroids. This would mean that athletes seeking steroids might also be exposed to a wide array of addictive drugs whose use is a criminal offence. It is also difficult to guarantee the quality of black market drugs, as the level of purity can vary significantly, and this is particularly true of steroids.

In addition to the 'steroid pushers' who ensure that the drugs are readily available even to teenagers in gymnasiums across Australia, there is evidence that steroids are being prescribed by a number of 'doctors' and sold by some pharmacists without prescription. A number of doctors, concerned that athletes might risk their lives taking drugs of dubious origin and in potentially lethal quantities, have felt that prescribing steroids to athletes is the lesser of two evils. Such doctors argue that while ever an athlete who is doping remains under their care, the side-effects of the drugs can at least be monitored and any deleterious impact upon, say, liver and kidney function can be assessed, thus minimising the damage that might otherwise be done.

In many countries there is at present no legal prohibition on the use of steroids, only on the sale or supply of them to others without prescription, such violations carrying a fine of around $A800 or six months in jail. The British government, on the other hand, is considering a move to classify steroids in the same category as hard drugs such as heroin, narcotics and cocaine. This being so, those who used or sold them could face criminal charges. This is an issue which is being hotly debated in many places around the globe.

The health risks of steroids

In regard to the health risks associated with steroids Dr Howard Nay of the Columbia University College of Physicians and Surgeons writes, 'The list of complications after using anabolic steroids is frightening and should serve as warnings for all but the foolish or suicidal.'[25] The most commonly documented of the major adverse effects of steroids relate to liver dysfunction and the formation of liver tumours and liver cysts. Other adverse side-effects for males include a reduction in the size of the testes, diminution of sperm quality and production, loss of libido (sex drive), and acne. For women, the lowering of voice, facial hair, and enlargement of the clitoris are not uncommon. Irreversible damage to the body caused by steroids has not only crippled and maimed our athletes—it has also led to their deaths. In one case a teenage American school footballer named Benji Ramirez died after having collapsed during a training session. It was the strong opinion of the coroner, Dr R. A. Malinowski, that steroids did contribute to the death of Ramirez.[26]

Why doping persists in sport

There are no easy answers to the question why, in the face of disqualification, public disgrace and considerable—even potentially lethal—health risks, athletes continue to dope. It is of course less than surprising that at the top level of competitive sports, especially in events where the levels of performance already mark the limits of human ability, athletes will turn to doping to gain that competitive edge over other athletes. It is well known that to gain that competitive edge some athletes are taking steroids in quantities twenty times greater than the recommended therapeutic dose. Speaking of steroids, Murray writes:

> Recommended therapeutic dosages for the oral forms (Winstrol, Anavar, Dianabol) vary from 2.5 to 10mg per day. A typical dosage for an athlete in training is 100mg per day and up, with as much as 400mg per day claimed. The oral forms, in conjunction with injectables like Decadurabolin, are often taken twice a week, rather than once every three or four weeks as recommended for therapy.[27]

In 1988 Dr Forest Tenant estimated that as many as one million athletes in the US alone are using anabolic steroids and current estimates indicate that Tenant's figures are conservative.[28] The statistics are in any case horrifying, and since Tenant's analysis of the situation, the revelation of unbridled steroid usage among teenagers has shocked the world. Researchers from Pennsylvania State University under the direction of Dr William Buckley in 1988 carried out a study of 3403 senior boys at 46 US high schools in which it was shown that 6.6 per cent had taken steroids. Extrapolating these figures Buckley suggests that somewhere between

250 000 and 500 000 adolescents in the US are taking or have taken steroids. It is all the more disconcerting to discover that two-thirds of the adolescents who have used steroids started doing so at age 16 or younger.

Given the young age of steroid users and the massive doses being taken, the health risks are all the more serious. It is suggested by some practitioners that young athletes who take heavy doses of anabolic steroids for 60 to 90 days should expect to die in their 30s or 40s. Dr Robert Goldman, chairman of the US Amateur Athletic Union's Medical Committee, laments, 'The scary part is, here we have the finest product of this country—our young people—and we're going to have an entire patient population developing diseases they never should have had in the next five or ten years.'[29] Nor is it the case that athletes are simply ignorant of the health risks involved. In a survey recently conducted by Goldman 198 world-class athletes were asked whether they would take a 'magic drug' which would guarantee them victory in any competition for the next five years. Goldman reports that more than half—103—said yes.[30]

What is it then that drives athletes to gain that competitive edge? What is it about 'winning' that makes it so important, even worth risking one's life for? When all is said, it would appear that the doping problem in sport is a facet of the drug problem in society. Continually seeking instant gratification, we have as a society turned to technological innovation, wherever it is found, as a short-cut to achieve our goals. In regard to drugs we have been seduced by the power of the pill as if the medicine cabinet was an armoury of magic bullets, to be used against the enemies of hard work and persistent effort. We have become progressively distracted as a culture from the way of nature to the way of the chemist. We have structured our society, our institutions and our technological innovations in ways which reinforce our craving for instant satisfaction and for the maximum of achievement with the minimum of effort. In essence, we have ourselves created a drug-culture, in respect of which drugs in sport are simply one expression.

There is perhaps no better example of this attitude and its universality than the extraordinary sales enjoyed by a book recently published in France, entitled *300 Medicines for Surpassing Yourself Physically and Intellectually.* Crammed with advice concerning the right drugs to take for everything from exam preparation to how to stand out in a crowd, 13 000 copies of the first edition and 20 000 copies of a second printing sold out within a few days. Despite protestations from the medical establishment that the book was an incitement to potential drug abuse, the book has to date sold more

than 100 000 copies and gone through five editions, and the pub-
lisher is having difficulty accommodating the continuing
demand.[31] The point is a simple one—not even the suggestion that
the book is a fake has served to deter the French reading public. If
drugs provide an easier way to satisfy one's desires than the route
provided by honest labour, so much the worse for honest labour.

In trying to teach our athletes that winning is 'not everything',
we have by our response to their 'losing' shown that we believe
winning is the only thing. The doping problem is thus from another
vantage a crisis of values. We live in a society in which 'not
winning' is tantamount to 'failing'. It is no accident of language
that we categorise competitors into two groups: 'winners' and
'losers'.

Once these values have become entrenched, it is no surprise that
social pressures of various kinds contribute to the doping problem.
The need to be successful is not an ego requirement peculiar to the
world of sporting competitors, but if the only way to succeed in
sport is to win, and if an athlete's sense of self-worth is wholly
dependent upon sporting success, it is perhaps understandable that
so many see the advantage of drugs as outweighing the costs.

Olympic nationalism only makes the problem worse, because
there the stakes are so much higher. To win is to succeed for the
coach, for the team, one's family and ultimately, for one's country.
Similarly, to lose is to fail not just oneself, but to fail the coach, the
team, one's family and ultimately to fail one's country. It is worth
noting also that spectators can be a source of tremendous pressure which athletes may find difficult to overcome without
performance-boosting aids. Athletes are expected not only to perform well—they are expected by the crowd *always to perform well*
and are usually expected *always to perform better.* The more they
are adulated as sporting heroes for their past successes, the greater
will be the pressure to continue to succeed.

The media also plays a significant part in placing pressure upon
athletes. The superstar status accorded by the media to successful
young athletes can create within them a false sense of identity and
self-worth. They may feel successful by reference not so much to
their actual sporting achievements as to the way which those
achievements are represented by the media. Media attention can
make or break an athlete. The media can create a gap between
actual performance-skills and expected performance-skills, thus
introducing a new dimension of pressure on an athlete apart from
the pressure of the competition itself. One way of dealing with this
pressure is to use performance-boosting drugs.

Last but not least, we are brought full circle to the matter of
sport as a form of big business. The financial and material rewards

associated with sporting success can be considerable. Promoters seek the best athletes to compete in their competitions; companies employ the elite athletes of sport to endorse their products, and a whole host of career opportunities in sales and marketing, not to mention sports commentating, await the best and most popular athletes. It is clear that the financial incentives associated with sporting success, with 'the win', serve to impose pressures upon athletes which in the end they find overwhelming. Many turn to doping as a way out. As the common saying in the US goes, 'You dope to cope'.

Legislation may help, but it is not simply the letter of the law, but the spirit of the law which needs to be enshrined. While we need to educate our athletes on an *international scale* to the dangers associated with doping, we need also to recognise the extent to which our current life-style covertly encourages the drug problem in sport. The real task is to articulate in educational terms a social philosophy and ethics of sport in which winning at any price is ultimately too high a price to be paid.

2 Senate standing committee on environment, recreation and the arts inquiry into drugs in sport
John Black

The Senate Environment, Recreation and the Arts Committee is one of the legislative and general purpose standing committees which is established by the Senate at the beginning of each session of Parliament. The functions of these committees are set out in Senate Standing Orders which state that committees 'shall be empowered to inquire into and report upon such matters as are referred to them by the Senate, including any Bills, Estimates or Statements of Expenditure, messages, petitions, inquiries or papers'. Standing Orders give the committees 'power to send for and examine persons, papers and records, to move from place to place, and to meet and transact business in public or private session'.

While it is normal for witnesses to be invited to appear before a committee, the power exists for witnesses to be issued with a formal summons to appear. Failure to abide by the summons could then constitute a contempt of Parliament, the penalties for which are a maximum of six months' imprisonment or a fine of 5000 Australian dollars for an individual, or a fine of $25 000 in the case of a corporation. The giving of false or misleading evidence may also constitute a contempt of Parliament as may the refusal to answer relevant questions. Senate committees are therefore very powerful bodies, particularly given their power to call for papers as well as for people. This is because the use of primary documentary sources can provide a very effective means of checking the evidence provided orally by witnesses at public hearings.

All the available powers of Senate committees were required to be exercised to the full during the inquiry into drugs in sport. This was initiated in a formal sense when on 19 May 1988 the Senate resolved that the following matter be referred to the Standing Committee on Environment, Recreation and the Arts: *'The use by Australian sportsmen and sportswomen of performance enhancing drugs and the role played by Commonwealth agencies'*.

At the time this reference was received the committee was already working on two other inquiries. Nevertheless, at the beginning of June 1988 advertisements were placed in national newspapers seeking written submissions on matters relating to the use of drugs in sport. The closing date for submissions was the end of July. At that stage I expected a short inquiry, one that could be completed within six months. As it turned out, this was a very optimistic view, and the issues surrounding the inquiry continue. Public hearings began on 11 November 1988 and by the time the 520-page interim report was tabled on 14 June 1989 the committee had received written submissions from over 60 individuals and organisations and had received or required to be produced to the committee a vast amount of documentary material from various organisations and individuals. There were at that stage 2158 pages of transcript of evidence taken in public and over 750 pages of *in camera* transcript.

The inquiry process attracted a lot of media coverage and public attention. This was partly because of the intrinsic interest of the subject, but it was facilitated by the decision of the committee to allow full television and radio coverage. This was done in order to emphasise the open nature of the inquiry and to make it clear that no cover-up was taking place. Another beneficial result of this decision was to increase community debate on the issues raised. This in turn meant that people who might not otherwise have been aware of the inquiry were encouraged to come forward and provide relevant information.

A detailed analysis of the evidence thus far taken by the committee is contained in the interim report. The report covers a wide range of matters and made twelve recommendations directed towards deterring the use of performance-enhancing drugs. Perhaps the most important recommendations related to the establishment of a completely independent Australian Sports Drug Agency (ASDA) to be responsible for all aspects of sports drug-testing in Australia. Other recommendations addressed matters such as the importation, prescription and supply of anabolic steroids and the licensing of gyms. While the report touches on a wide range of

issues, I have been asked to address one subject in this paper—
although a very broad one—the scope and limits of the drug
problem in sport.

The use of drugs to enhance performance, while not always
illegal, is nevertheless banned by most sporting organisations. Athletes caught using drugs on the banned list are likely to be subject
to penalties of one sort or another, and will certainly have their
reputations tarnished. This means, inevitably, that sound quantitative data on the extent of the problem is difficult if not impossible
to come by. However, the powers possessed by a Senate committee,
together with the protection afforded by parliamentary privilege,
can go some way towards overcoming the barriers to truthfulness
that would otherwise exist.

On the basis of the evidence available to it, the committee finally
concluded that the abuse of performance-enhancing drugs by
sportspeople is widespread and is accepted as normal practice
among some groups. Drug abuse is more prevalent in some sports
than in others but it appears that performance-enhancing drugs are
used in virtually all sports, at all levels and by both amateur and
professional sportspeople. Most alarming of all is that drugs are
known to be taken by children, in some cases with the knowledge,
if not the encouragement, of their parents.

In reaching this conclusion the committee made use of three
distinct kinds of evidence. These were first, anecdotal evidence;
second, the analysis of drug tests performed on athletes; and third,
the results of the Survey of Drug Abuse in Australian Sport. Each
of these types of evidence has problems of reliability but, taken
together, the limitations of each are compensated for by the
reliable features of the others.

In considering the anecdotal evidence it is important to remem-
ber that it was taken under oath and that witnesses were made
aware of the serious penalties that can apply to anyone trying to
mislead a committee of the Parliament. Morever, some of the
witnesses who appeared before the committee did so only after the
issue of a formal summons, and did not volunteer their evidence.
Rather than provide a detailed analysis of the evidence, which can
anyway be found in the report, I will provide some quotes to give
the flavour of the evidence heard by the committee.

Mr Kelvin Giles, who has been a British National and Olympic
coach and who was first head coach of the track and field at the
Australian Institute of Sport, told the committee that: 'At the very
elite level—I am talking about the top 10 or 20 in the world— 95
per cent of them are taking [drugs]'.

Also at the elite level, the Australian Olympic Federation (AOF)
told the committee that the 'use of anabolic steroids is claimed to

be reasonably widespread'. In a minute to the executive directors and secretaries of national sports federations in June 1987, the AOF Secretary General noted that 'the AOF is concerned that practices prohibited by the IOC are prevalent'.

At the non-elite level, Dr Millar told the committee that while there may be 3000 athletes using anabolic steroids in Sydney alone, in Australia there would be only 200 top athletes who would benefit from using the drugs. This confirmed other evidence that the majority of users are at lower levels, often recreational sportspeople. This is possible because of the ready availability of these substances, particularly the anabolic steroids. Mr Ian Childs told the committee, for example, that: 'If you wanted to train now and go on steriods, we could nominate you a gym where you could literally walk in, put your money on the counter and you would get steroids. You would get them that day, or you would get them the next day.'

The ready availability of anabolic steroids is one reason why they, along with other performance-enhancing drugs, are being abused by children. The committee heard of weight-lifters as young as 10 who were taking anabolic steroids and Dr Gavin Dawson described the situation in bodybuilding where: 'This sad situation has descended to junior levels where, because of peer competition, pills are being popped as if they were competing against the Communist countries'. The abuse of performance-enhancing drugs by children is a matter of particular concern to the committee and we will follow up this issue in some depth.

The impression received by the committee from the large amount of anecdotal evidence it received is that the use of performance-enhancing drugs, particularly the anabolic steroids, is not only a common and accepted practice, but is in many cases seen to be necessary for involvement in the sport. There have even been suggestions, which we will be following up as the inquiry proceeds, that in a few sports the officials may see the use of drugs as necessary because they are themselves involved in their distribution.

The results of drug tests carried out on athletes may suggest that the anecodotal evidence tends to exaggerate the use of performance-enhancing drugs. However, the problems involved in using drug test results to access the level of drug usage are amply demonstrated by the case of Ben Johnson. According to his coach, Johnson had passed seventeen post-race drug tests in 1986 and 1987, even though he was taking anabolic steroids during this period.

Some in-house Australian drug testing also seems to have been just as inefficient. The committee heard evidence that a weight-lifter was tested at the 1987 Moomba weight-lifting competition and found negative for drugs. At the same time this weight-lifter, by his own admission, was bulking-up on a course that involved ingesting up to 32.5 mg a day of Lonavar (oxandrolone) and receiving injections of Sustanon, a mixture of synthetic testosterones, and gonadotrophin. As you might expect, the committee intends to follow-up this case in some detail.

Extrapolating from drug test results to the proportion of participants taking drugs has the following defects:

* Testing has focused on competitions, and athletes can adopt drug usage regimes to ensure they are drug-free by the time of competition.

* Substances such as blocking agents and masking agents, as well as diuretics, have been used to decrease the effectiveness of drug testing.

* The testing system may itself be corrupt.

In fact, some of the most telling evidence for the widespread abuse of drugs, certainly at the elite level, comes from the corrupt practices employed in drug-testing.

Mr Kelvin Giles told the committee how the selection of athletes for testing could be based on first finding out whether they were drug-free. He said:

When I toured Europe before I retired in 1986 from track and field coaching, taking Australian teams and other teams from around the world through Europe to the major meetings ... I would very often be asked by the meet director or one of his aides, 'Are all the members of your group okay for drugs testing? Would you mind submitting to drug-testing?' ... It was obvious that, if you said, 'We do not want to be tested; they will be found positive' they would not test you.

Even when athletes have been selected, urine collection procedures may not always be as carefully managed as they should be. To demonstrate this I will quote from a letter written by an Australian Institute of Sport coach to the then Australian Athletic Union and which was obtained by the committee.

At the Birmingham competition I accompanied [an athlete] for a dope test ... No attempt was made to identify the person presenting for the test. Had I tried I am sure I could have passed myself off as [the athlete].
[He] was unable to pass a specimen at the time of his reporting to the officials. He was then allowed to leave the testing room and told to report back in one hour. During that time he was not supervised by any testing official. On reporting back ... [he]

objected to being required to pass a specimen into a container
which was not sterile and which had been used previously by other
athletes . . .
    Finally when passing the specimen, [he] was not strictly
supervised. He was able to go into a cubicle on his own, a situation
that could allow attempted abuses of the procedure.

The committee's report also describes in detail an incident in
which an Australian sporting official, at a meet in Europe, initiated
an attempt to substitute a urine sample from an athlete by that of
another. In this particular case it seems that neither athlete would
have tested positive, but the incident does say something about the
perceived widespread use of drugs. I should also point out that one
whole chapter of the committee's report was devoted to describing
the many deficiencies in the drug-testing program carried out by
the Australian Institute of Sport. This is not to say, of course, that
athletes at the AIS were taking performance-enhancing drugs
(although some admitted doing so). The point is that the testing
program carried out at the AIS cannot be used in any way to prove
that drugs were not being used.

The selection and testing procedures at the AIS were carried out
in such a careless way that no action could have been taken, even if
an athlete *had* tested positive. For example, an analysis of AIS
drug-testing files showed that four athletes were drug-tested several
days *before* they were randomly selected for their respective tests.
Someone at the AIS must have had a very effective crystal ball for
this to happen.

The committee examined 99 specimen identification forms on
the AIS files. Less than 10 per cent of these met the required
standards of documentation. Some showed no chaperone, or male
athletes with a female chaperone, for example. Only ten contained
the signature of both chaperone and an area supervisor, in accordance with accepted procedures. Two of these ten tests involved a
delay between selection for testing and the time of giving a urine
sample of longer than the allowed 48 hours.

A charitable view of the way the AIS approached the collection
of test samples is that it seems to have been one of having a
drug-testing program for appearances' sake, with little attention
paid to its effectiveness.

Even once samples have been collected there is a possibility of
interference and the committee received evidence of samples being
lost. This need not always be deliberate of course, and I noted with
interest a report in the *Sydney Morning Herald* of 4 August 1989
that seven test kits of urine, taken as drug test samples from
athletes at the Australian marathon on 23 July, had disappeared
from an Australian Airlines flight.

It is clear that for all the reasons stated the results of drug tests give a very limited idea of the extent of drug usage. Positive tests show only the tip of the iceberg and there is some justification for the view that only those who have foolish have been caught. A further problem with reliance on drug test results to estimate the size of the problem is that testing has been directed largely at elite athletes, and, as already discussed, the greatest number of users can be found among the non-elite group.

I should say here that this situation will change for the better once the recommendations in the committee's report have been fully implemented and there is a regular, large, completely independent testing program involving targeted and random testing, as well as competition testing.

The third type of information on the abuse of performing-enhancing drugs comes from the 1983 Survey of Drug Use in Australian Sport (Australian Sports Medicine Federation, 1983). This was based on a simple questionnaire distributed by the sporting organisations of 31 sports to 14 200 sportspeople who were asked to complete the survey anonymously. The final analysis was based on a sample of 4064 sportspeople.

The survey is a wealth of valuable information but is inevitably out of date and concluded that there appeared to be a significant problem with drug use in Australian sport. This is particularly so in that more respondents to the survey said that it was their intention to use anabolic steroids in the future than had admitted to using them in the past. In other words, the survey found that the problem was going to get worse. It was for this reason that the committee recommended that the national program on Drugs in Sport conduct a survey, based on the methodology of the 'Survey of Drug Abuse in Australian Sport' to help define the extent to which banned drugs are abused by amateur and professional sportspeople at all levels, and of all ages, and to determine the attitude of these groups towards performance-enhancing drugs in order to see if there has been any change since the previous survey.

I have described in very brief outline some of the evidence taken by the committee which led it to the inescapable conclusion that the use of performance-enhancing drugs by Australian sportspeople is widespread. What I have not addressed is why this is a problem.

One of the most striking features of the inquiry to date has been the inability of most witnesses to put forward logically consistent arguments as to why drugs should be banned in sport. Even those opposed to the use of performance-enhancing drugs seemed to think it quite reasonable for athletes to take very large quantities of vitamins, inosine and other tablets, as well as other food supplements, to improve performance. Twenty, 30, even 50 tablets a day seems to be not unusual and accepted as normal by athletes, their coaches, doctors and others involved in sport. And these tablets may well be supplemented by vitamin injections or injections of substances such as adenosine triphosphate (ATP). It is not a trivial question to ask why these substances are accepted but the use of anabolic steroids or other substances on the banned list is not.

The committee made its position on this matter quite clear. It opposed the use of performance-enhancing drugs because of their potential to damage the health of those using them. There are serious health risks associated with the use of these substances, often long-term, and many not appearing until several years after the drugs have been taken. These effects are often not known or understood by the sportspeople concerned. Moreover, the behavioural changes caused by some of these drugs (particularly anabolic steroids and stimulants) can cause a lack of judgement and increased aggression on the part of those taking them. This can result in doped sportspeople becoming a danger to their competitors.

I would like to emphasise that the committee rejected the argument that doping should be banned because the use of drugs is unfair. Although this is still one of the most commonly used arguments it has no plausibility at all.

Sport is not fair in the sense of this argument. Enormous inequalities of opportunity exist for those trying to compete at both the national and international level. The advantages in terms of funding, facilities, expert advice and support in everything from diet to sports medicine and coaching, vary widely from one country to another, and within countries. It is noticeable, for example, that many athletes from poor and developing countries move to other countries to take advantage of the better facilities and support being offered, and it is not unknown for Australian athletes to move overseas because of the better opportunities they find there. The playing field has always been uneven and, with recent advances in knowledge and techniques, is getting more so.

Those individuals and organisations who complain that the use of drugs is unfair do not seem concerned about these other sources of inequality, and seem able to accept that an injection of human growth hormone is wrong, but that to take amino acids purportedly to increase the body's production of growth hormone is permissible. Similarly, it is considered fair to train at high altitudes to increase blood haemoglobin levels, but wrong to try to achieve the same end by blood doping. Recognition that the problem is one of health is important in community education on this matter.

The dangers associated with the use of drugs are now being recognised by the general public. A survey carried out by Insight

Research in Queensland, for example, found that 93 per cent of the adults surveyed supported a ban on the use of performance-enhancing drugs. Most of the respondents to the survey believed that athletes who took drugs regularly were endangering their health. When asked to rank the danger from 'a lot' to 'not at all', 65 per cent of the sample agreed with the former statement, only one per cent with the latter.

The results of this survey are important and encouraging. This is because one of the major factors contributing to sportspeople, particularly elite sportspeople, taking drugs, is the attitude of the society in which they live. Community attitudes and the pressure to win placed on athletes by the media and politicians can be as important as the opportunity for personal reward in tipping the balance on an athlete's decision to take drugs. General recognition of the health risk involved in the use of drugs may well influence the way athletes behave.

The committee's report made twelve recommendations, of which the most important was that an independent Australian Sports Drug Commission be established to carry out all sports drug-testing in Australia. The Insight Research Survey already referred to found that 86 per cent of respondents supported this idea, while only 9 per cent opposed it. The recommendation has, of course, been accepted by the government and the commission has been established. It may be worth pointing out here that the community debate stimulated by the committee's inquiry also led to a number of actions to further reduce the availability and use of performance-enhancing drugs being taken during the course of the inquiry. These were listed in a document that was incorporated in the Senate Hansard of 14 June 1989.

The reception accorded to the committee's interim report led to the address from September 1989 of the black market in performance-enhancing drugs and the use of drugs in certain high risk areas such as power-lifting. We also took evidence on the health risks of performance-enhancing drugs from people who had themselves experienced some of the serious side-effects of these substances. Other issues addressed in more detail were the use of these drugs by children and their use in professional sport. The intensity of the investigation into professional sports will depend upon the willingness these sports have shown to subject themselves to the scrutiny of the Australian Sports Drug Agency (ASDA).

To sum up. There has been a widespread and serious drug problem in Australian sport. However, with greater community awareness of the nature of the problem, and with the very positive response to the recommendations made by the Senate Committee, it does look as if there is a possibility of making real progress.

With the implementation of the drug testing program recommended by the committee, and with similar action being taken
by other countries, we should be able to develop an environment in
which no athletes will feel themselves disadvantaged if they say
'no' to sporting drugs.

3 The future of the Olympic movement
Arnold Beckett

In my opinion, the three major problems facing the Olympic movement now, and in the future, are the influences of politics, of professionalism and of drugs. In many ways, these three aspects are inter-related, but my emphasis in this chapter will be on the policies and measures adopted by the IOC Medical Commission and the various international federations of sport in response to the problem of drugs in sport.

In the last decade, the Olympic movement has been beset by problems resulting from the withdrawal from Olympic Games of various member countries, in compliance with political agendas that have little to do with sport itself. In Montreal in 1976, Moscow in 1980, and again in Los Angles in 1984, various countries attempted to make political points by their failure to appear. Of course the Commonwealth Games has also been beset by similar problems.

When Lord Killanin (the then President of the IOC) was challenged by the press in 1980 at the Winter Olympic Games in Lake Placid concerning the damage international politics was doing to sport and particularly to the Olympic Games, he acknowledged serious problems but opined that these would be overcome. He used the opportunity, however, to focus attention on the problem of drug misuse in sport, which he stated would destroy sport completely unless the matter could be brought under control. The President of IOC in 1991, Juan Samaranch, has also been very forceful in pointing out the danger which drug misuse constitutes for sport.

The rise in the importance of the involvement in professional sports has also had its impact upon the Olympic movement. However, the change from the rather hard line during the presidency of Mr Brundage to the more moderate line taken by Lord Killanin and then by Mr Samaranch, has shown the Olympic movement to be responding positively to the changing circumstances affecting sport at the top level.

Drug misuse in sport—the world awakening

Doping in sport has occurred for many decades, but the dramatic increase started in about 1960 as society as a whole came to believe increasingly that there were drugs available to deal with most ills, diseases and problems. Inevitably, sport as part of society became caught up with this drug culture and some competitors, coaches and doctors began to look upon drugs as aids in taking shortcuts to success. Attention focused on this problem in 1960 at the Olympic Games in Rome when three Danish cyclists were taken to hospital and one, Jensen, died. His death was associated with the use of stimulant drugs. At the 1964 Olympic Games in Tokyo there was an attempt to start drug testing at the Games. At these Games the International Federation of Sports Medicine passed resolutions on the problem and some members played important roles in mobilising opinion in the Olympic movement. Prince Alexandre de Merode of Belgium had just been elected a member of the IOC, and organised a meeting with David Brundage, then President of the IOC, the result of which was the creation of the present IOC Medical Commission in 1966.

Philosophy and practice of dope control

The IOC Medical Commission was given a number of tasks, one of which was to draw up plans to try to deal with drug misuse in sport. It was first necessary to provide a coherent philosophy and to delineate the borders between permissible use of drugs in treatment and inappropriate and obvious abuse (see figure 3.1).

The IOC and the IAAF medical commissions, although recognising that the misuse of drugs in attempts to enhance performance in sport contravened the basic ethics of fair play and fair competition between competitors, concentrated their main emphasis on providing clear rules which could lead to action if contravened, i.e. the pragmatic approach. The evidence was already available that not all doctors and coaches had the welfare of the

---

Figure 3.1 Why should some drugs be classed as doping agents?

Moral argument

Their use contravenes the essence of the sporting contest: the matching of the natural capabilities of the participants.

Pragmatic arguments

- Competitions should involve competitors, not pharmacologists and physicians
- Competitors should not be used as guinea pigs
- The use of some drugs can cause aggression and loss of judgement—hazards to other competitors, spectators and officials
- The misuse of drugs sets a bad example to young people
- Competitors can become dependent on certain drugs

---

competitors under their care as their first priority. Pressures to succeed at all costs were in evidence in top-class sport. Those involved in trying to produce a coherent philosophy and plan realised that if competitions in sport were allowed to degenerate into competitions between pharmacologists and physicians with competitors being used as guinea pigs, and receiving potent drugs for non-medical use, then inevitably there would be more deaths in sport from drug misuse and sport would be set on a path that would lead to ultimate disaster.

It was decided to draw a firm line between permitted use and unacceptable use in sport by producing a list of banned classes of compounds and giving sufficient examples in each case to demonstrate the purpose of the control envisaged (figure 3.2)

To produce a definitive list of banned compounds would only have led to the use of related compounds for which similar pharmacological actions have been demonstrated, and even to the use

---

Figure 3.2 IOC Medical Commission policy on dope control

- To prevent the use of those drugs in sport which constitute dangers when used as doping agents
- To prevent drug abuse with the minimum interference with the therapeutic use of drugs
- To ban only those drugs for which suitable analytical methods could be devised to detect the compounds unequivocally in urine (or blood) samples
- To ban classes of drugs based upon the pharmacological actions of members of the classes but not to attempt to produce a complete list of banned drugs

---

of compounds not marketed as drugs for medical use; this of course was already occurring in society in the use of designer drugs. Therefore, the first lists and the present ones contain under each class of compound the words 'and related compounds'. This has often led to criticism that the Commission has not produced a definitive list.

The IOC Medical Commission decided to include only banned classes for which suitable analytical methods were available to identify unequivocally in urine the compounds and their metabolites. This, as we will see later, was altered to deal with certain problems. The IOC Medical Commission was well aware even in 1960 of the misuse of anabolic steroids and had the evidence of their misuse in cycling in 1968 at the Olympic Games in Mexico City; however, because certain analytical methods were not then available, this class of compounds was not banned until 1975.

When the rules were introduced by the IOC in 1968 and testing at the Games commenced, there were some reporters who attacked the testing on the grounds that such testing constituted an interference with the rights of the individual. They argued that a person was entitled to do anything to himself in his attempts to achieve success, and therefore he should be allowed to use drugs, even if that use meant death. The rights of the individual, therefore, were strongly stressed and it was argued that already there were enough rules and regulations without introducing any additional ones.

Within about one year, however, opinion was overwhelmingly in favour of action to prevent the escalation of drug misuse. It was realised that the majority of competitors were in favour of action. It was realised that those on drugs could constitute hazards to other competitors who were not using drugs. Thus, the drug-free person might suffer harm as a result of drug-taking over which he had no control.

The various aspects of dope control that were addressed by the IOC Medical Commission are shown in figure 3.3.

The selection of athletes must be seen to be fair, whether it is by random selection or places. At the Olympic Games, the first four in each singles event are tested and at random tests are conducted on competitors in heats and finals.

The control of the urine collection is very tight—it must be established by observation that the sample comes from the individual under test. The sample is divided into A and B so that if the laboratory reports an adverse finding in the A sample, the B sample can be analysed before appointed delegates. The laboratory analysis is carried out on the coded sample and the identity of the

Figure 3.3 Aspects of dope testing

- Selection of athletes to be tested
- Control of sampling
  Bottles
  Codes
  Urine collection
  pH measurement
  Subdivision of sample
- Transport and control of samples
  Sealing
  Codes
  Laboratory receipt
- Reporting of results
- Repeat analysis on duplicate sample
  Method
  Observer
- The use of control 'positive samples'

competitor is thus not known to the laboratory. Reports are made to the chairman of the Medical Commission who can decide to identify the individual.

Positive 'control samples' are fed into the system to act as part of the quality assurance scheme.

Laboratories are accredited for the purpose of this work by the IOC Medical Commission.

The IOC and its Medical Commission were prepared to take their international role in the fight against escalating drug misuse but it was essential to have the support of the international federations of sport and of national governmental authorities. It was equally important to have public awareness of the problems and public support for the proposed action.

Public awareness of the magnitude of the problem became increasingly apparent over the last decade and especially during and after the Olympic Games in Seoul. The disqualification of Ben Johnson and then the revelations during the Dubin inquiry in Canada (figure 3.4) focused world attention.

In all, there were ten positive doping cases at the Seoul Olympics, of which five were weight-lifters (figure 3.5). The International Weight-lifting Federation (IWF) carried out its own investigation suspending the Bulgarians and Hungarians for two years and the Spaniard for six months. The Olympic athletes themselves made a declaration (figure 3.6)

Figure 3.4 Evidence given by Doctor Astaphan at the Dubin Inquiry. Canada, 24 May 1989

Dr Astaphan stated that he had:

- injected Johnson with his knowledge and consent with anabolic steroids between 50 and 60 times since early 1984;
- prescribed TESTOSTERONE to Johnson;
- prescribed HUMAN GROWTH HORMONE (HGH) to Angela Issajenko, the leading Canadian woman sprinter. (Said Astaphan: 'I think she was sharing it with other athletes'.);
- got 14 bottles of HGH for CHARLIE FRANCIS—the coach of most of Canada's leading sprinters.

The competitors had also been acting at Olympic level to stop sport being destroyed by drug misuse by emphasising that coaches and doctors were involved as much as athletes. Sebastian Coe, the Olympic gold medallist, spoke on behalf of many athletes at the Olympic Congress at Baden-Baden in 1981: 'We consider this (doping) to be the most shameful abuse of the Olympic ideal: we call for the life ban of offending athletes; we call for the life ban of coaches and the so-called doctors who administer this evil.'

Sports federations outside those involved in the Olympic Games are also acting. Government bodies are calling for action because

Figure 3.5 Weight-lifters who tested positive for banned substances at Seoul Olympic Games, 1988

Bulgaria   —   Mitko Grabley gold medal
           —   Angel Guenchev gold medal
Hungary   —   Andor Szanyi silver medal
           —   Kalman Csengeri
Spain   —   Fernando Mariaca

The above were disqualified from the Games and lost their medals.

Figure 3.6 The Seoul declaration of Olympic athletes. 27 September, 1988

We share the ideals laid down in the Olympic Anti-doping Charter and urge all partners in sport throughout the world to implement the programme.

We call for the establishment of unannounced random testing for athletes in training and competition on an international basis.

We call for a full inquiry of each doping case, to review the involvement of all concerned, including the athlete, coach and administrators, and call for severe punishment for those found guilty.

We call for more education for athletes, coaches and administrators to teach the dangers of performance enhancing drugs and thus to prevent future doping infractions.

politicians have begun to realise the implications for their countries of escalating drug misuse in sport, recognising that sportsmen and women act as important role models for teenagers.

The Council of Europe acted in 1984 and a European Antidoping Charter was agreed and similar action was taken by Socialist countries. The first permanent world conference on antidoping in sport was held in Ottawa in June 1988; the second conference was held in Moscow in October 1989. In 1989, the Council of Europe recognised the lead being taken by the IOC in adopting the International Olympic Antidoping Charter and welcomed it setting up an independent doping control team for out-of-competition testing.

In Barcelona in 1990, an agreement for the prevention of doping in sport was made between the IOC and the international summer sports federations. The agreement was aimed at harmonising IOC and international federations' antidoping rules, procedures and sanctions. The Commission and the federations agreed:

• to harmonise as rapidly as possible their antidoping rules and procedures, both for controls during, and out of, competition (unannounced tests);
• to adopt each year as a basic minimum the list of banned classes and methods of doping as established by the IOC Medical Commission and as relevant to each sport;
• to harmonise the sanctions for violations to the antidoping regulations in accordance with the recommendations made by the IOC and to ensure their application at national level;
• to recognise sanctions given by another international federation;
• to use the laboratories accredited by the International Olympic Committee, as well as the IOC's mobile testing laboratory for all major international competitions and out-of-competition testing;
• to cooperate fully with the national Olympic committees, national federations and governmental organisations in order to fight against the trafficking of doping substances in sport.

IOC Accreditation of laboratories for doping control

The laboratories accredited by the IOC for doping control must meet demanding standards. The areas covered by these standards are summarised in figure 3.7. Laboratories are helped to achieve these standards and then finally for accreditation they have to analyse, in front of a designated scientist, ten samples of which the Doping Sub-Commission has full analytical data; ten out of ten results must be correct and the appropriate documentation and information leading to these decisions must be provided.

Figure 3.7 IOC Scientific and technical guidelines for laboratories engaged in doping control

Objectives

Comprehensive operational standards
Best available technology—reliability and accuracy
Continuous update to guidelines

Facilities

Environment, space, utilities, safety, storage
Instruments
General facilities

Personnel

Directors
Responsibility for quality assurance and quality control
Scientific, technical and non-technical staff

Quality assurance and quality control

Information, collection and record-keeping requirements

After accreditation, laboratories have to meet the proficiency testing program and reaccreditation procedures (figure 3.8). Sometimes accredited laboratories fail to meet the standards of reaccreditation and they are then not allowed to carry out final tests for international events until they again reach the required standards according to a specified procedure.

The IOC Medical Commission has done all in its power to ensure that correct analytical aspects and laboratory procedures underpin the objective information on which decisions are made about doping. Because advances are continually being made and new problems arise which must be solved, the laboratories must be involved in research if they are to function effectively. To date, it seems to be those laboratories which do not function in this way have problems in meeting standards. It is advisable for such laboratories also to be involved in the appropriate fields of drug

Figure 3.8 IOC-accredited laboratories: annual reaccreditation procedures

Analysis of 10 control samples—reporting of results

Provide a fully documented report including raw data

Complete a questionnaire—re personnel, instrumentation, space etc

Proficiency testing program

Analysis of 4 urine samples every 4 months (excluding the reaccreditation period)

Provide results and documentation

Figure 3.9 Doping control: principal goals

Laboratory

To determine unequivocably the presence of drugs of the banned classes in samples of urine presented to it as coded samples.

To obtain correct results on the 'B' samples.

To report the findings to the Medical Commission, and to no-one else.

Medical Commission

To identify the person providing the urine sample i.e. from the code.

To consider the results provided by the laboratory.

To discuss the reason for the presence of drugs and/or metabolites in the urine sample from the competitor.

To decide whether the presence of the drug constitutes a case of doping.

To decide what shall be its recommendations for action and report to an executive group. i.e. Executive of the IOC or committee of national or international federation.

---

metabolism, pharmacokinetics, bioavailability etc. and to publish their work so that it is subjected to international scrutiny.

The role of the IOC Medical Commission must be to ensure that the analytical methods used in the accredited laboratories in dope control testing are published in reputable scientific journals, so that the basis of the tests is available for international examination by other experts in related scientific disciplines. If quantitative or semi-quantitative limits are to be set as part of the control, then the appropriate documentation which led to the specified limits must be published and thus available for public scrutiny. The system must not only be fair and supported by scientific data, but be seen to be so by other scientists who might wish to challenge the situation.

Functional goal of IOC-accredited laboratories

The functional goal of laboratories is to obtain objective results and report them to the Medical Commission, which then should decide on whether a positive doping case is involved after they have examined all the information available. The careful steps taken between initial drug detection and the possible imposing of sanctions are listed in figure 3.9. It must, however, be stressed that the IOC has always stated that the deterrent and educative aspects of doping control are of paramount importance, and that punitive measures are taken only to that end.

Figure 3.10 Samples analysed by IOC-accredited laboratories during 1988
(Answers received from 20 laboratories)

	Number of samples	Number of negative samples	Number of analytically positive A-samples	Percentage
Competitions with national competitors only	16 925	16 497	428	2.53
Competitions with international competitors	13 706	13 379	327	2.39
Major international championships	4 930	4 790	140	2.84
Samples collected out-of-competition	10 140	9 919	221	2.18
Checking of competitors prior to major championships	1 368	1 331	37	2.70
TOTAL	47 069	45 916	1 153	2.45

The statistical data emerging from analytical results obtained by laboratories are of obvious importance. Some of these results are shown in figures 3.10 and 3.11. It should be recognised that in most cases the results are obtained in those who know that testing is occurring. Thus the 2 to 3 per cent of positive results only represent the tip of the iceberg of drug misuse in sport (See also chapter 5 for more details.).

IOC and international federations of sport

The close relationship between the IOC and international federations of sport plays an important role in the overall fight against doping in sport. Many federations have accepted the leadership role of the IOC with regard to classes of banned drugs, procedures, sampling, penalties, appeals, etc. This is important because the need for harmonisation is great. For instance, it seems unfair that some sports ban the use of antihistamines for treatment of hay fever and other allergies because the drugs have some sedative effects. Is it correct for a national organisation to attempt to ban a competitor for life for having a caffeine concentration above the proscribed limit when the level could be exceeded by drinking unwisely too many cups of coffee in too short a time?

It should be recognised that the fight against drug misuse in sport will only be supported by legislators and decision makers

Figure 3.11 IOC-accredited laboratories: substances identified in positive A-samples, 1988

Stimulants — 420		Anabolic steroids — 791	
Pseudoephedrine	140	Nandrolone	304
Phenylpropanolamine	109	Testosterone	155
Ephedrine	48	Stanozolol	89
Cocaine	42	Metenolone	60
Amphetamine	23	Methandienone	54
Methamphetamine	14	Methyltestosterone	33
Methylephedrine	8	Oxandrolone	22
Caffeine	6	Boldenone	19
Phentermine	5	Dehydrochlormethyl-testosterone	16
Amfepramone	4	Oxymetholone	12
Heptaminol	4	Mesterolone	11
Pemoline	3	Clostebol	6
Cropropamide	2	Drostanolone	4
Crotetamide	2	Formebolone	2
Chlorphentermine	1	Fluoxymesterone	1
Etafedrine	1	HCG	1
Fencamfamine	1	Methandriol	1
Fenfluramine	1	Trendbolone	1
Methoxyphenamine	1		
Nikethamide	1	*Diuretics — 57*	
Pentetrazol	1		
Phendimetrazine	1	Furosemide	35
Phenmetrazine	1	Hydrochlorothiazide	17
Prolintane	1	Triameterene	2
		Bendroflumethiazide	1
Narcotics — 58		Bumetanide	1
		Canrenone	1
Codeine	35		
Propoxyphene	6	*Beta-blockers — 8*	
Dextropropoxyphene	4		
Dihydrocodeine	4	Propranolol	7
Morphine	4	Metoprolol	1
Hydrocodone	4		
Normethadone	1	*Masking agents — 19*	
Oxycodone	1		
Pentazocine	1	Probenecid	19

when the rules, regulations and penalties are considered to be reasonable by a consensus of informed opinion.

The IOC has stated clearly its rules and regulations and has tried to give guidance to federations with regard to penalties when rules are infringed. The recommended sanctions of the IOC Medical Commission are:

- Anabolic steroids, amphetamine-related and other stimulants, caffeine, diuretics, beta-blockers, narcotic analgesics and designer drugs: 2 years for the first offence, life ban for the second offence

• Ephedrine, phenylpropanolamine, codeine etc. (when administered orally as a cough suppressant or painkiller in association
with decongestants and/or anti-histamines): a maximum 3
months for the first offence, 2 years for the second offence, life
ban for the third offence.

The Commission recommends that before a final decision is made
on a particular case, a fair hearing be granted for the athlete (and
possibly the other persons concerned). Such a hearing should take
into consideration the circumstances (extenuating or not) and the
known facts of the case. During the hearing, it is also recommended that the head of the IOC accredited laboratory who
reported the result be consulted.

The Commission also recommends to sports authorities that
even more severe sanctions have to be taken against all persons
other than the athlete involved in the doping case if the guilt of
such persons can be unequivocally established.

The IOC has demonstrated its determination to act against those
who have been involved with the competitors in a breach of the
doping control rules. It has shown its desire to arrive at correct
methods and rules by the involvement of experts who are not
members of the Medical Commission. It has stressed the need for
basic research and set up the International Olympic Association
for Research in Sports Medicine in 1982 for this purpose, although
perhaps it is now necessary to broaden and make more effective
the basis of the research commitment.

Some federations have held important conferences, in addition
to the IOC, to deal with the various aspects of the problem, including an attempted objective appraisal of the problems and dangers
involved in drug misuse and the dangers which are likely to occur
as new drugs and procedures become available; moral and philosophical aspects are also now beginning to command attention.

IOC banned classes of drugs and future problems

The IOC list of banned classes and methods specified by the IOC
in April 1990 is shown in table 1 of chapter 6. Under each class,
the IOC gives examples to indicate the nature of the banned class.
In a sense, the banned classes are always out-of-date as the race for
newer, better, less detectable substances continues apace. The
misuse of hormones is a developing serious problem in the attempt
to circumvent present controls. The IOC Medical Commission
therefore, has recently introduced a ban to deal with the changing
circumstances. Professor Brooks of the UK, based upon his own
research, has put forward a proposal for establishing scientifically

when human chorionic gonadotrophin has been misused. However, full validation of the test is necessary before it is possible for action to take place. And new challenges will emerge as Growth Hormone-releasing factor becomes more widely available.

Erythropoietin (EPO) as a possible substance for blood doping is already a reality; the problem was addressed in the 2nd IAF World Symposium on Doping in Sport held in Monaco, in 1989. Suitable analytical techniques to combat this misuse, however, are not currently available.

The IOC must keep abreast of the new changes but it is well recognised that drug-testing alone will never solve the increasingly difficult problems of drug misuse in sport. Scientific advances involving recombinant DNA techniques and gene splicing are occurring at such a pace that the IOC has a limited time available to change the attitude of all those involved in sport so that drug misuse becomes unacceptable to all. Unless all countries and individuals can be assured that other countries and individuals are not misusing drugs or techniques to give an unfair advantage then the problems posed by the use of hormones and non-drug techniques will overwhelm the dope control system.

Society has failed totally to deal with the problem of drug misuse, which is undermining the social fabric in many countries. The record of sport in the area of drug abuse is not good. The question is can sport rid itself of the evil of drug misuse quickly enough, so that those involved in sport can constitute role models to influence society as a whole? The IOC will require cooperation from international sports federations, from national sports federations, from competitors and coaches, and doctors and officials and politicians and parents and teachers and the media, if it is going to ensure that sport fulfils this role.

The alternative advocated by some of allowing the use of any drug in any amount and the use of any techniques in the attempt to improve performance in sport is surely the alternative of despair —and a complete negation of the ideals of the Olympic movement.

NOTE: All tables and figures in this chapter are derived from documents and proceedings of 10C Medical Commission.

4 Is there a place for drugs in the performing arts?

Elizabeth Toohey

I would like to preface this chapter by pointing out that the Australian Ballet like most ballet companies, is quite insular. Our odd working hours and extensive travelling schedules limit our social contacts with others outside the ballet world. Hence my comments on the use of performance-enhancing drugs are confined to my experience of that world.

It would appear that most athletes use drugs either for the building of muscle or for their effect as stimulants. In our profession, on the contrary, the maintenance of a constant standard and level of fitness is paramount, so that continued good health is our first priority. All dancers are aware of diet and how to get maximum energy from the food we eat, and we realise that a decent meal is going to do us far more good than using drugs for energy or hype.

The basic difference between the attitude of dancers and sportspeople lies in the fact that dancers do not compete. While sportspeople will work each day to build towards a special race or event, dancers have to keep their physical peak for months on end because we perform every night. Basically we compete against ourselves, always trying to improve our technique, but we don't try to break world records for the most pirouettes ever performed or the highest leap ever jumped on stage. For us incredible fitness and grace are equally important aspects of performance, never forgetting that the performance itself is indeed an art form.

Each dancer has his/her work load laid out in terms of a specific number of performances of any given role and must consistently produce the goods at these engagements. There is also a problem that if another dancer becomes injured one may be called on, on some occasions at very short notice, to replace them. Consequently we have to be continually at performance peak; for 'the show must go on!' So without the use or help of drugs such as amphetamines how do we sustain such high standards for up to and sometimes in excess of 12 hours a day, 6 days a week, 48 weeks a year and in my case 12 years up till now? It takes a little while for the individual dancers to realise what suits them best, but by and large we maintain a healthy lifestyle and cope with our more specific problems, e.g. personal motivation, which relate to getting the most out of our individual performances.

I will start with the attitude of dancers who take the spotlight and show how differently they approach a special performance. Certain roles in particular ballets are renowned as the most difficult as far as stamina is concerned. The duration of such ballets is approximately two and three quarter hours, and within that time there are two 20-minute intervals. For the gentlemen a perfect example is Romeo in *Romeo and Juliet.* Romeo rarely leaves the stage and has to contend with difficult solo work and intricate fight scenes, culminating in the scene in which he kills Tybalt. The role is draining, both physically and emotionally. To boot, there are the many pas de deux with Juliet, when he must lift her as if she were as light as a feather.

For women a similar role as far as stamina is concerned is Kitri in *Don Quixote.* Kitri is on stage most of the time. The role is very gutsy and the choreography requires an enormous amount of energy and technical skill from start to finish. I might add that during the two 20 minute intervals the dancer doesn't sit around doing nothing. It is always at this time that one has to change costume and hairstyle and make sure everything is in readiness for the next act. The most a dancer will eat or drink then is about half a glass of Staminade.

Obviously these roles can't be danced every night by the same dancer and the maximum one could expect would be three performances a week—for optimum results two performances a week would be perfect but sometimes this is impossible.

With natural adrenalin I find I always have enough energy to through a difficult role provided I've prepared myself well during the day. This entails not over-exerting the muscles and eating a reasonable meal about four to five hours before the show. A lot of dancers find that their main problem is trying to calm themselves down. The way I find most effective is to practise breathing control and to maintain a very positive outlook about the performance ahead. It is very easy to ponder over the many things which might go wrong during the performance. Considering the technical skills and timing required, one often has the feeling, 'I've only got one opportunity to show the audience and prove to my peers I can do it'. This feeling can lead to the dancers actually faltering, or becoming quite upset about tiny aspects of their performance.

The best way to approach an evening of technical difficulties is to treat the day as normal, not to become preoccupied, and to keep one's mind off anything that might cause anxiety. I believe there is no need for any sort of drugs whatsoever. In fact if we added chemicals to our body we wouldn't be in nearly as much control, and that is so important not only for one's own performance but for one's partner's. Timing must be perfect, and partners must feel a rhythm and rapport with each other.

There are also dancers who need to hype themselves up. They treat the day of a performance as something special. They sit quietly and contemplate what they will be performing that evening so that they can go on stage and forget about technicalities and inhibitions. This is the way they find works best. Without a doubt all dancers have to cope with nerves in one way or another, and it is just a matter of time before individual dancers find the way that works best for them.

Obviously the Corps de Ballet face a different set of problems because they perform every night. Making each performance look fresh even though it may be the twentieth performance in three weeks demands a discipline of its own. These dancers face less of a technical challenge each night on stage than do the soloists but without doubt each member of the Australian Ballet puts 100 per cent into each performance, knowing that their colleagues are counting on them.

I would like to speak for a moment about my overseas experience. Although my overseas tours have taken me to various countries, I have spent the majority of my time in the Soviet Union. This I consider a great privilege as the Soviets are renowned as the greatest dancers in the world. I am honoured to say that David McAllister and I are the only Australians ever to be guests of the two greatest companies in Russia—the Bolshoi in Moscow and the Kirov in Leningrad. We have also been guest artists with four other major companies from the Baltic States to Southern Georgia.

In Russia the basic attitude to performing is somewhat different from ours in the west and there are various reasons for this. The Ballerina dancing in the evening performance will come in and do morning class but only just as much as she feels necessary—nothing too strenuous, just loosening the joints and stretching the muscles. She then may have a rehearsal at which her partner and the conductor are both present. In this case she will just walk through the performance, talk about *tempis* and perfect little details of the *pas de deux* or solos involved. Then she may have a light massage, something to eat, and she will rest. She'll prepare herself early, do her performance and then she will have the entire following day off. This is unheard of in Oz.

The reason dancers can be treated this way is that most Russian companies have an abundance of dancers e.g. the Bolshoi has 300 and the Kirov has 250, so we must consider them elite in comparison to most other companies in the world. At any one time, a number of dancers are capable of performing the major roles, so that a generous rotation of performance and rest days *is* possible. The Russians specialists also tend to be more versatile than our top dancers, so that the leading Russian dancers perform only once or twice a fortnight. Hence they tend to perform up to and into their fifties, because they haven't had such a strenuous workload in the early part of their career.

I have said earlier that there is no place in a dancer's life for amphetamines or anabolic steroids. The latter deserves comment. The building of muscle is essential to every dancer, but it is the type of muscle one builds which is most important. A male dancer can't look like a weight-lifter. His body must appear to be totally in proportion.

A male's physique has to be as graceful in its own way as a female's. So a man builds long, lean muscle—primarily without the use of weights—and builds strength through the specific exercise that dancers must do every day. Artificial drugs would add bulk that would not be aesthetically right in a dancer, despite any advantage in strength such drugs might give him. Some of the strongest dancers with whom I have ever danced actually don't look strong because they lack muscle bulk. This is because of the way dancers are taught when they first learn the *pas de deux*. It is not so much strength as fine coordination that is required for a man to lift a girl directly over his head, simply with one hand, and to hold her there for as long as the audience deems fit. This is unlike weight-lifting where the athlete lifts the bar-bell over his head, holds it there for a short period of time, and then releases the weight.

The male dancer's plight is in the hands of the audience. At the end of a difficult *pas de deux* where the man has been constantly lifting the girl, dancing and leaping himself for up to ten minutes, he then has to lift the girl above his head with one hand and stay there until the audience finishes clapping. It's a moot point then whether a standing ovation is a good or a bad thing. If the audience stops clapping after 35 seconds, well and good, and he can bring his partner down—but if they are bravoing and applauding he has to keep her there till they stop. So coordination is the key. It is a target skill for a male and is the thing we work on the most from our first *pas de deux* to our last. The woman can help a great deal by holding herself in such a way that it makes the lift as light and easy as possible.

Anabolic steroids, therefore, are unnecessary and to my knowledge have never been used within the Oz Ballet. Amphetamines, too, are out because we need to calm ourselves down before a performance. This isn't to say that dancers don't use or even at times abuse drugs. The most commonly used drugs within the ballet world would have to be anti-inflammatories and aspirin. From my experience aspirin is not abused but the former is.

All dancers at some stage in their career will have to perform with a certain degree of injury for a couple of reasons—either because they can't be replaced in a specific role or because the injury is not severe enough to stop performing altogether. Drugs are prescribed by our company physician after he has diagnosed the nature of the injury and they give the dancer almost immediate relief. The most common injuries for dancers include knee, back and ankle strain, all of which have a certain amount of tendonitis involved, which makes it necessary to take anti-inflammatories.

It is sometimes tempting to continue to use this drug even after a few days when the inflammation should have gone down. Sometimes, because of the relief felt by the dancer, he or she can start to become dependent on the drug and that can be a dangerous thing. When we are given the drug we are told to take them for a few days and see how we feel, and only to take them when we feel it's absolutely necessary. I have known of some dancers who took Naprosyn—the most common anti-inflammatory for dancers a couple of years ago—for twelve months. Consequently after they stop taking the drug they are faced with all sorts of other problems.

Aspirin for pain relief is something we all take at times. It is not abused but I feel is worthy of comment as it is commonly and openly used, especially when dancers who are in pain cannot be replaced and have to perform.

Pain-killers aside, it is a fact that dancers drink and dancers smoke—basically for the same reason as most others. We have a drink after a long hard day or to wind down after a performance and those who smoke do so on a social basis. Really there is no place in the performing arts for the type of drugs that are such a problem in competitive sport.

There have been articles and books written about the use and abuse of drugs and alcohol in the performing arts in America, specifically the use of cocaine, and insinuations that artistic directors have fed their dancers amphetamines to hype them up for a performance. What individuals will succumb to is a very different thing from what is common practice. And if an individual wishes to gain notoriety and blow such incidents out of proportion by publication, that is a matter of choice.

I have read Gelsey Kirkland's *Dancing on My Grave*, and if any credence is to be given to her account, it is my opinion that the problem lies with her. The dance world can't be blamed at all.

5 Fair play: ethical issues of doping in sport
Vernon Howard

'Equal conditions for all' is the deceptively simple definition of fair play to be found in the *Oxford English Dictionary*. A recent publication of the National Collegiate Athletic Association in the US declares, 'The use of drugs to enhance athletic performance violates the very principles of fair competition'.[1] Assuming that such 'principles of fair competition', nowhere spelled out in the NCAA pamphlet, are rooted in the idea of 'equal conditions for all', I shall go to the philosophical heart of the matter. What do we mean by 'equal conditions'? Are such conditions specifiable, realisable, and inflexible, as the NCAA document tends to assume? Or are they regulative, relative, and variable with time and circumstances?

These are tough questions made even tougher by the widespread use of drugs in sport to kill pain or to enhance performance. If so many athletes are taking drugs, why should drugs constitute an 'unfair advantage'? In other words, why is drug use a violation of fair play? This is quite a different question from, What are the potentially harmful side effects of such drug use? The one is a question of principle; the other a question of fact. Most public discussions run the two queries together, assuming that because the drugs in question may (or do) have harmful side-effects, they constitute an unfair advantage (presumably on the part of those willing to take the medical risks). The NCAA pamphlet and most opinions on the topic that one encounters in the popular press and media are cast in exactly that moralistic tone. 'Drugs in sport are evil and dangerous. Period. So let's eliminate 'em. Period.' Notwithstanding the seriousness of the practical problems (which I in no way doubt or denigrate), such black or white thinking masks the larger conceptual and moral issues involved. As a philosopher and onetime competitor long out of touch with the sports scene, I am entirely dependent upon others' factual knowledge of the physical and psychological effects of drug use in sport. I cannot pretend to definitive judgements on the factual questions. The best I can offer is the sketch of a conceptual framework for the question of principle within which appropriate medical and training decisions might be made—a logical geography, as it were, of fair play and drug use. I should be satisfied if what I have to say resulted in a better appreciation of the full force of the medical information as it impinges upon the moral and philosophical issues of fair play.

Equal conditions for all

Equal conditions for all is the sports equivalent of the general moral principle of equal justice for all. Equal justice for all implies that the same justice applies to everybody regardless of class, origin, race, gender, and the like: in effect, no exceptions and no special privileges. This suggests by analogy that fair play construed as equal conditions for all means the same conditions should apply to all competitors—no exceptions, no special privileges or advantages save those we call 'handicaps' designed to even out the very performance differences that would otherwise ensue if the competitors were evenly matched.

But what does it mean for the conditions to be the same? Runners in the same race may wear different makes of shoes and may have trained in quite different ways. No matter. Times from different races run at different dates and places are compared directly. Again, no matter so far as the record books are concerned. Yet if one of the runners is discovered to have taken anabolic steroids, we cry, 'Foul! Unfair advantage! OK to change your shoes but not your chemistry.' So, to repeat, which conditions are relevant to fair play and which are not? And why?

Such conditions may be either intrinsic, peculiar to the athlete himself or herself, or extrinsic, peculiar to the environment in which the athlete is competing. For example, we are unlikely to complain about the systematic use of certain types of mental imagery, 'stress management', or meditation to enhance training and performance; whereas we do complain about anabolic steroids, less so, perhaps, about amino acids, and even less (but sometimes) about vitamins.

By the same token, breakthroughs in equipment can trigger controversy. If my memory serves me correctly, a flap arose in the 1950s over the springier synthetic vaulting poles, which seemed to give unfair advantage over those competitors still using the less flexible bamboo poles which created a noticeable gap in the record books. Similarly, American baseball fans argue over the comparability of records set before and after the advent of the so-called 'live ball'. In both instances the new equipment prevailed, the one for unleashing a potential to reach new vaulting heights, the other for making the game faster in an impatient age. Not at all controversial, however, were those coveted Australian Kangaroo-skin flats and spikes of the same era, alleged to give any runner or jumper a long leg-up. So the line between fair and unfair conditions cuts across conditions both internal and external to the athlete to encompass every aspect of the competitive environment including its scientific study.

The latter point deserves underscoring; for we must also deal with long-term advances in knowledge of biochemistry, of biomechanics, and of genetic predisposition in sport.[2] It could well happen that certain kinds of knowledge and its dissemination (or lack thereof) became the unfair advantage of the future, far outpacing the emergence of new equipment or today's reliance on pain-killing and performance-boosting drugs. For example, Laval University exercise physiologist, Claude Bouchard, declares that 'Within ten years, we hope to have a battery of gene probes that will identify the genes associated with the gifted athlete. The probes are used to identify, but now for a limited number of genes, the ones that we know are useful in certain movement. With that research, we can get the selected [children] into early training programs.'[3]

Bouchard's focus is not on genetic engineering or selective breeding but rather on genetic screening for specific athletic potential. Even so the prospects he outlines for the near future are but one step away from genetic engineering for athletic purposes. What then becomes of fair play? Competition among super men and women especially bred and reared (or 'merely' screened) for the purpose? Ben Johnson, the deposed Canadian sprinter, suggested as much at the Dubin inquiry in Toronto in May 1989. Blithely ignoring the moral issue of harmful drug side-effects, he recommended that sports competition be segregated as between those competitors taking performance-boosting drugs and those who don't. However abhorrent such a prospect may be to some of us, it could come to pass in some quarters (and probably will, since the medical technology is within reach). One envisions sperm banks for basketballers, gene pools for gymnasts, indeed, a whole new

'industry' of sports eugenics. As for the rest of us genetically rele-
gated to the mongrel leagues, it would surely be unfair to pit us
against the thoroughbreds. Old Dobbin was never any match for
Citation even if he ran himself to death in the effort.

I raise this spectre of the modern Colosseum merely in order to
emphasise two points about fair play. First is the fact that whatever
we have to say about fair play is embedded within a larger moral
context definitive of what we think ought to be the case ideally
even if it isn't or cannot be fully realised. (More on ideals of fair
play and doing things 'naturally' later on.) Fair play among thoroughbreds is one thing; whether we should undertake genetic
screening for athletic purposes is quite another, though both are
moral issues.

If, in the spirit of Kant, we view moral principles as assuring the
treatment of human beings always as ends in themselves and never
as mere means, then genetic screening may appear to run against
the moral grain.[4] Yet one can imagine arguments to the contrary:
that genetic screening could contribute to the diagnosis and prevention of injuries, to the improvement of training methods, to the
early recognition of one's best potential—a kind of physical apti-
tude test. The point is that moral principles require interpretation
and critical argumentation at all levels of their application, not
stereotypical enforcement according to fixed precedent.

A second purpose of these ruminations on the modern Colosseum is to emphasise the fact that 'equal conditions for all' is a
highly relative notion, more a desideratum, an ideal, than a set of
absolute restrictions unaffected by sports medicine, science, and
technology, not to mention what one might call the 'social pathology' of sport—the examination of our culture's obsession with
athletic prowess. Present day doping is but one aspect of this much
bigger socio-ethical picture.

Having unearthed all these complexities, I should now like to
change the subject. I want to talk about a less well know counter-
part to doping in sport; namely, doping in the performing arts.
Analogues are both interesting and enlightening, and lead to a
useful distinction.

The ups and downs of doping

As a performing artist—a classical singer—for ten years of my life,
I had a problem: stage fright, especially in formal recitals and
auditions, less so in well rehearsed performances or dramatic set-
tings. I often felt at a disadvantage when auditioning. My cooler,
less nervous colleagues always seemed to do better than I; that is,

they performed closer to their potential for the part than I because they were better able to control, or simply did not experience, the shaking knees, roiling diaphragm, dry throat, and diffused concentration that afflicted me whenever I had to compete for a role.

Imagine then my consternation, my chagrin, when I recently read a (to me) compelling article in *The New England Journal of Medicine* by Alan H. Lockwood, MD entitled 'Medical Problems of Musicians'[5] in which he reports that two drugs called propranolol and nadolol effectively eliminate the physical, and therefore, most of the psychological, symptoms of stage fright. In medical terminology, Lockwood perfectly describes my symptoms.

> Performance anxiety is a syndrome characterised by nervousness, fear, tremors, tachycardia, shortness of breath or 'tight' breathing, sweaty palms, dryness of the mouth, nausea, and an urge to micturate. It takes little imagination to see how these symptoms, attributable to excessive adrenergic tone, can severely impede a high-level musical performance. Tremors interfere with bow control and fingering among string players, and tight breathing and a dry mouth affect wind instrumentalists and singers. The presence of these symptoms increases the anxiety level and may lead to further decrements in performance.

A more vicious cycle for the performing artist, in my instance, auditioning artist, cannot be imagined. Nor could I imagine that pharmaceutical help was available, for I'd always been told that tranquillisers and alcohol had damping effects as bad if not worse than the effects of stage fright itself. Until, that is, I read Lockwood's recommended treatment (p. 225)

> Beta [adrenergic]-blocking agents are clearly indicated in the management of severe performance anxiety. For many, this may be the only treatment necessary. For others, such drugs may be a useful component of a multiple-approach stress-management program in which beta-blockade can be used to demonstrate to the patient that high-level performance is possible, thereby enhancing self-confidence sufficiently so that routine use is not necessary.

If such drugs had been available to me, and I was given reasonable assurance that no serious side effects would occur, I'd have taken them—not, I hasten to add, to enhance my performance beyond its normal potential, but to be able to sing up to it.

Here, in this personal anecdote and from the medical information given in Lockwood's paper, we have the makings of a useful distinction; namely, that between equal performance opportunity versus unequal performance opportunity. That is, we may distinguish between those drugs that give one an equal advantage versus those that give one an unequal advantage, between those drugs that eliminate an impediment and those drugs that actually boost performance. To try to clarify this distinction, let us assume for the sake of argument, that two drugs were available to me in my predicament: propranolol to control the disruptive symptoms of stage fright and another, fictional one, that I shall call 'vocalonol'—a drug of no suspicious side-effects that will enable me to inspan my nasal pharanx, develop and flex my aryvocalis and diaphragmatic muscles beyond all my previous levels of performance. And consider these test findings about vocalonol: 85 per cent of respondents who took vocalonol reported marked improvements in their 'mechanical' abilities: no breaks over the entire vocal range, greater timbral and dynamic control, extended endurance, amplified resonance, and no strain in the upper registers. The felt effects were described as comparable to what nonprofessionals might experience singing into a closet full of clothes and then singing in the shower. What is more, vocalonol is thought to increase one's aural sensitivity to, and mental concentration upon, specifically musical phenomena. And since vocalonol has never been known to interact aversely with propranolol, it is truly the singer's dream drug.

Should I take it? That depends. Note that propranolol allows me to sing up to my normal potential, increasing my capacity to sing as well as I normally can by eliminating certain preventive conditions (cf. Scheffler,[6] on preventive conditions). Vocalonol, on the other hand, enables me to sing far beyond my 'normal', one might even say, my 'natural' potential—a bit like having a bionic voice. A long standing taboo in opera and classical singing proscribes mechanical amplification on grounds of distorting the 'natural' timbre and projection of the human voice. By contrast, popular singing without the aid and 'working' of a microphone is virtually unheard of.

So what? Isn't the idea to get the best performance possible out of everybody? Well, that's just the point. If I'm auditioning among others who do not have access to vocalonol and have no idea that I'm on the drug (I neglected to mention that it is also hideously expensive), I would seem to have an unfair advantage. Why? Because some other singer of greater beginning ability than I stands to be cut out, who, if he used vocalonol, might sing even better than I. The same might apply to my use of propranolol too were its effects not generally know and were it not available to other, similarly afflicted auditioners. Still, with propranolol all I seek is equal advantage—the opportunity to do my normal, 'natural' best.

General knowledge and access are clearly moral factors in this equation. Without them, I would seem to have an unequal advantage with either drug but particularly in my use of vocalonol. The situation differs somewhat in my use of propranolol; for there, although I have an unequal advantage over other stage frightened auditioners, I have no special advantage over other performers. You might say that my performance is 'liberated' by propranolol—like killing a headache with aspirin before an examination—but not artificially enhanced. Propranolol puts down certain preventive conditions to my singing potential; vocalonol artificially 'amplifies' my singing potential beyond its normal limits.

Therefore, while we may distinguish between drugs of equal versus unequal opportunity, perhaps even criteria for sorting drugs into one or the other category, whether a particular drug constitutes an equal or unequal advantage depends upon the details and context of each case. In other words, applying such a distinction, however logically or medically drawn, is a piece-meal, 'bottom-up' interpretive matter, not a matter of 'top-down' categorial enforcement.

Shortly, I want to come back to the notions of what is 'natural' or 'normal' versus what is 'artificial' or 'enhanced'. They heavily qualify what counts as equal conditions for all, and therefore, the very idea of fair play. But for the moment, let me reiterate an earlier distinction. There is a difference between the moral grounds for rejecting the use of a drug in sport or elsewhere because of its real or suspected harmful side effects and rejecting that same drug because it seems to give an unfair advantage. As mentioned at the outset, because of their frequent coincidence, we tend to run the question of fact and the question of principle together. The question of fact is easier, if not easy, to handle ethically.

Even if some artists or athletes are willing to risk the medical consequences of a suspect drug, that is no moral case in their favour; for then, they are treating themselves as mere means to an end: turning themselves into singing, running, or vaulting machines. For example, *Sports Illustrated*,[7] commenting on the Ben Johnson scandal during the Seoul Olympics, quotes a source as saying that Johnson was receiving 'incredible amounts of this stuff' [anabolic steroids]. However, he [the source] said, Johnson's advisers did not even do blood profiles on Johnson to see if his liver and his kidneys were capable of handling the steroids. 'It was like he was a racehorse. A commodity', said the source. Such individuals are caught in a Faustian bargain wagering their souls, talents, and bodies for success at any cost. Vince Lombardi, the late American football coach, is often quoted as having said, 'Winning isn't everything, it's the only thing'. I set that next to Nietzsche's sardonic remark that man would rather have the void for purpose than be void of purpose.

One can only blink in dismay at the equally pernicious social 'side-effects' of any art or sport deliberately bent to the ends of blind ambition, crass commercialism, jingoism, or politics. And what of the example of the Ben Johnsons et al. to others? As the Existentialists have long reminded us, what we do establishes a precedent of behaviour, a principle for others to follow (without, of course, getting caught). *Sports Illustrated*'s sources quote Dr Jamie Astaphan, Johnson's doctor in St. Kitts, as telling them[8] 'that the Americans and the Soviets did not know how to administer drugs to enhance the performance of their athletes without the drugs being detected, and that his "idols" in sports medicine were Bulgarian team doctors who were expert at this deception.' By such deceptions and false 'idols' do laudible risks for noble ambitions get twisted into lamentable means to sordid ends. In May 1989, Dr Astaphan testified at the Dubin inquiry in Toronto where he described the prevailing ethos among world-class amateur and professional athletes as, 'If you don't take it, you won't make it.'

To come back to the question of whether performance-boosting drugs are always unfair in principle, consider the following variation on an earlier example. If propranolol and vocalonol are both generally available, safe, and known to be, what is to distinguish them morally from other, uncontested aids to vocal training and development? I venture to say, very little. Why not get the very best singing out that can be gotten by all safe means? Let all who need it take propranolol and all who want it take vocalonol. No need to bargain with the devil for the voice of your dreams; bargain with DuPont instead!

Similarly, if you could take a drug of no suspected harmful side effects that would make you brilliant, give you the insights of genius, enable you to express ideas with extraordinary power and depth—even knowing that others might do the same and better— why deprive you of that experience, even if it is by some measure unnatural? Call it Pharmaceutical Grace of Enlightenment. And if the mere prospect of this sub-Faustian bargain brings to mind the Bible's words, 'What doth it profit a man . . . ', I can only think to reply with the DuPont Corporation's laconic slogan, 'Better things through chemistry.' The logical point here is that the moral case for safe boosters is stronger where the element of competition is replaced, or at least strongly qualified, by 'loftier' humanitarian goals, say, of self-improvement, greater knowledge, or artistic achievement. I venture that if sport were seen more in this

'Plympian' perspective, so also would our attitudes positive and negative towards performance-boosting drugs be altered. But, and the 'but' is a big one, delayed side-effects are exceedingly difficult to detect in advance. On the positive side, who would have thought ten years ago that aspirin would be prescribed as a preventive medication for heart disease? That Avon bath oil would prove an effective insect repellant? On the negative side, who would have thought ten years ago that AIDS might be the risk of promiscuous sex? Or 40 years ago that soldiers present at atomic bomb tests would later exhibit unusually high rates of cancer? Even knee bends have a bad reputation nowadays! We have to balance off what we think we know against the wages of gain, and that inevitably involves risk. Life itself is a constant risk,[9] but that is no excuse for Faustian bargains where we or our young people are concerned. Reasonable risks and honest mistakes are one thing, deliberate exploitation of oneself or others is quite another.

On being normal and natural

The normal thing is often just the done thing—everyday, typical practice—or it may be the natural, uncontaminated thing. On the one reading, performance-boosting drugs are quite 'normal' because common; on the other reading, such drugs are 'abnormal' because unnatural and contaminating. But what is it to be natural and uncontaminated? It will come as no surprise to anyone that this seemingly simple question has no simple answer.

From natural ability, to natural foods, to having a natural manner, to the injunction always to follow nature, the terms 'nature' and 'natural' exhibit alarming shifts of meaning. Far from being meaningless, 'nature' and 'natural', like 'creativity', 'imagination', and other portamento words, carry so many meanings willy nilly as to be unfissible. Yet so much rides on what is considered natural, according to or against nature, in this context that throwing our hands in the air at the mere mention of the terms will hardly suffice. So what are we to do? As a general strategy, Ronald W. Hepburn[10] suggests the following:

> In a particular philosophical context the sense in which nature is being used can be brought out most clearly by insisting upon the question 'What is nature (or the natural) being contrasted with in this context?' In one group of cases the natural is contrasted with the artificial or conventional ... The artificial and conventional are seen as interferences, modifying by an alien causality the characteristic patterns of behaviour. In the sphere of human nature

... it is by no means easy—if, indeed, possible—to delineate a human nature free of interferences, left to itself. Organism and environment, individual and cultural climate, are in ceaseless interplay.

Setting aside all metaphysical queries about uncontaminated human nature, as well as medical questions about drug side-effects, what is nature (or the natural) being contrasted with in this context, in the context of doping in sport and elsewhere? My guess, based solely upon what I read and hear, is that a common use of the label 'unnatural' refers to the aforementioned drugs of unequal opportunity, not to any and all drugs as one might hastily suppose. Thus, the unnatural would include the safe vocalonol as well as the unsafe anabolic steroids (the latter being doubly proscribed as unfair and unsafe). This leaves what I have called drugs of equal opportunity—propranolol, aspirin, and the like—relatively unsullied unless discovered to be unsafe or, in particular cases, to be abused. This once again illustrates the pincer-like logic of the situation: principles of fair play on the one hand, particular instances of drug use on the other, and our attempts to bring them together to make a judgement.

Where does this leave such performance-boosting practices as blood doping, carbo-loading, and vitamin dosing? Since technically these are not drugs, they may appear to lie outside the range of the unnatural. But in fact they do not; and that fact in turn forces us to broaden the concept of the unnatural to include practices of unequal opportunity including, of course, drugs. In other words, the line between a natural (in this context, equal) and an unnatural (unequal) advantage cuts across the lines, however drawn, between what is and what is not a drug and what is or is not a safe drug. Again setting aside the issue of side-effects, some practices and some drugs alike are seen to be natural or unnatural depending upon whether they give an equal or an unequal advantage.

I hasten to add that this is but one of many meanings attached to the natural/unnatural dichotomy. Yet another use of the noun phrase, 'natural advantage', for example, refers to exactly the opposite of equal opportunity when predicated of individuals; as, for instance, when we say Jones has a natural advantage in training or (or presumed native ability) over Brown in this or that sporting event. But because it is a natural advantage, it is permissible.

Here the importance of precedent comes into play; for whether a given practice or drug is viewed as giving an unfair advantage largely depends upon how widely known and established it has become. Carbo-loading, for example, is commonplace among distance runners nowadays, blood doping far less so. The latter remains more in the realm of 'alien causality' than the former; but is that likely to remain so as athletes desperately search for undetectable, presumably safe alternatives to anabolic steroids? I can only raise the question, the point being that changing practices and new knowledge alter the content, if not the principle, of our thinking about fair play—what shall count as being fair or unfair.

Aside from the fact that the natural/unnatural dichotomy admits of more and conflicting meanings than could ever be encompassed by a single definition, the terms are also used evaluatively. That is, the natural/unnatural dichotomy is affectively loaded. As Hepburn remarks, 'the natural, for instance, may come to be more highly esteemed than the artificial and conventional, as the spontaneous or the basic is contrasted with the laboured and derivative. The preference may be reversed, however: the natural can be taken as the mere raw material, the unfinished and preparatory, requiring artifice to complete and crown it.'[11]

In other words, to describe something as a natural process, action, or reaction could be neither to esteem it or to demean it. Generally speaking, nowadays to describe something as natural is to praise it as somehow 'uncontaminated', unmolested by 'alien causality'. It was not always so. J. S. Mill, for one, in his Essays on Nature remarks that, 'Nearly all the things which men are hanged or imprisoned for doing to one another, are nature's every day performances.'[12] Accordingly, his advice where human nature is concerned is 'not to follow but to amend it.' Clearly, we evoke Mill's connotation of the term whenever we condone any kind of training or educational procedure in order to shape 'raw' human nature; and just as clearly we evoke the sacrosant notions of nature and the natural whenever we condemn a practice as 'violating' human nature. To do so in the context of sport is, by extension, to violate the principle of fair play as well. But where do we draw the line between shaping and violating human nature?

As with controversies over sexual perversion, abortion, suicide, and euthanasia, we need independent criteria for determining the unnatural, contaminating, abnormal, or violating practices; but of course there are none generally agreed upon, unless one is already committed to a particular metaphysical, theological, or moral point of view.[13] So, when conflict arises, rather than searching for possible common ground in such controversies, or admitting the influence of changing conditions on the application of principle, one tends, rather, to fall back upon one's presumptions about what is natural, unnatural, or supernatural in order to defend one's judgements. The typical result is more shouting than sense.

To complicate matters even further, among those presumptions certain analogies and images of nature and the natural have floated (perhaps flooded would be the better word) down to us through the ages. These range from Aristotelian biological metaphors of preordained growth (the proverbial acorn), to medieval portraits of nature as God's handiwork (and Divine Will), to 17th and 18th-century cosmologies of nature as a mechanical-causal system, to 19th-century evolutionary metaphors of self-transformation and survival of the fittest, to 20th-century pantheistic images of ecosystems (cf. Hepburn, 1967, and Wollheim[14] on the thorny problem of which aspects of nature to select for moral guidance). From a logical standpoint, whenever arguments of principle and their right application rest on such loose footings they inevitably become wars of conflicting world views.

Can impasses of this kind be avoided, at least practically diminished? They can, but only if the participants in such controversies are willing to change their terms of discussion from what is natural or unnatural to what specifically is at stake. That means, first, taking Hepburn's advice to heart always to ask what exactly is being labelled natural or unnatural in this specific context and why. So, for example, if the issue comes down to what constitutes an equal or unequal competitive opportunity, stick to that. If it comes down to the real or suspected risks of harmful side-effects of certain drugs or training practices, stick to that.

Second, as soon as possible, abandon the idiom of loaded labels for the idiom of inquiry and justification. For example, if you think using vocalonol to enhance vocal performance constitutes an unfair because unnatural advantage, ask yourself, why is it unnatural? Because the resulting performance is beyond one's usual limits? What's wrong with that? Because one could not do it unaided by the drug? What's wrong with that? Because others may not have access to vocalonol, or because one just prefers the sound of 'unenhanced' voices, like preferring unamplified singing?

What this sequence of queries suggests is that labels like natural versus unnatural, like good and bad predicated of art works, function more as invitations to inquiry rather than as concluding judgements, more as challenges to the understanding than as resting places for belief. A genuine interest in Mozart's *Don Giovanni* is hardly satisfied by the pronouncement, 'It's good'. Neither does the pronouncement, 'It's unnatural', go very far toward settling any question of the fairness or unfairness of doping or other practices in sport. As starting points for discussion and inquiry, however, 'It's good' or 'It's unnatural' are as good as any.

Conclusion

Can one consistently, let alone practically, maintain such delicate moral balance on the question of doping and fair play as I have been trying to do in this essay? Frankly, I doubt it, but I cannot be sure. But of this I am sure: in the face of moral indecision, the better part of prudence as well as of wisdom is not to close fist on any of these issues, but rather to keep them open in ways that leave them accessible to rational discussion and inquiry, and just as importantly, revision in light of new knowledge, new options, and changing attitudes. By no means, however, am I recommending rampant relativism or a posture of anything goes. Rather, I am recommending that case-study interpretation as well as scientific and philosophical inquiry accompany our efforts to enforce conditions of fair play every step of the way.

I began by elucidating the notion of fair play as equal conditions for all, relating the latter to the larger principle of justice. I went on to argue that equal conditions for all is a relative, not an absolute ideal like truth in science, a desideratum, not a set of absolute restrictions independent of time, circumstances, knowledge, or sports technology and medicine. From there, I went on to suggest a distinction between drugs, and more generally, practices, of equal and unequal opportunity. At the core of that distinction is the difference between whatever eliminates certain preventive conditions and whatever enhances one's performance naturally or unnaturally. Of course, the very idea of what is natural or unnatural is moot for all the reasons aforementioned despite the common currency of that way of talking about such issues as doping in sport, abortion, euthanasia, and the like. So I recommended abandoning that idiom as quickly as possible in any controversy for the more specific, precise idioms of scientific and philosophical inquiry as more likely to yield useful results. Finally, I suggested that with a shift from exploitative to more humane values, even performance-boosting (safe) drugs may have a morally legitimate role in sport and elsewhere.

Allow me to end on a personal note. In the back of my mind as I began to write this essay was something like the atmosphere of *Chariots of Fire*, an atmosphere not unlike my own competitive days. Sadly, as I ruminated further on the complexities of fair play and doping in sport, I realised that the relatively simple conditions of the past no longer existed. My knee-jerk responses were obsolete. That fact, however, gradually became a challenge to me; a challenge to re-articulate what is it to be a fair and honest competitor in an age of biochemical technology. If I have done no more than raise certain perplexities to the level of philosophical examination, I am satisfied.

6 Biochemical aspects of substances banned by the IOC

David A. Cowan

With the multitude of powerful medications available today, the West has come to expect that there is a 'pill for every ill'. People also think that many of these agents can act as ergogenic aids to put one into a supra-normal position. We are in the age of the 'chemical man'.

Given the plethora of pills available, one may find it difficult to distinguish ethically why some tablets e.g. vitamins, amino acids, minerals, are considered as permissible whereas other tablets may be restricted in their use e.g. amphetamines. Indeed the fact that they are frequently difficult to distinguish in appearance, often being white in colour, does nothing to simplify the matter. When one considers that sportspeople may require supplementation of the water soluble vitamins, for example, to meet their daily requirement then it is not surprising that sport does not wish to restrict their use.

The simplest way to determine what is and what is not permitted in sport is to look at the regulations. The International Olympic Committee provides the common base for all Olympic sports and indeed for most international federations.

Table 6.1 shows the current IOC's list of doping classes and methods. It is divided into three groups: 'doping classes', which comprise the main groups of substances whose administration is banned by most international federations; 'doping methods', which include blood doping and pharmacological, chemical and physical manipulation. 'Classes of drugs subject to certain restrictions' covers additional classes which may be controlled by certain sports

Figure 6.1 International Olympic Committee   List of doping classes and
methods—April 1990

DOPING classes

• Stimulants

• Narcotics

• Anabolic steroids

• Beta-blockers

• Diuretics

• Peptide hormones and analogues

DOPING methods

• Blood doping

• Pharmacological, chemical and physical manipulation

CLASSES of drugs subject to certain restrictions

• Alcohol

• Marijuana

• Local anaesthetics

• Corticosteroids

NOTE: The doping definition of the IOC Medical Commission is based on the banning of pharmacological classes of agents. The definition has the advantage that also new drugs, some of which may be especially designed for doping purposes, are banned.

e.g. alcohol in shooting, or whose use may be permitted under specially controlled conditions e.g. corticosteroids.

A full list of IOC-banned doping classes and doping methods, and of drugs subject to certain restrictions is to be found in Appendix 6.1

Before discussing what the drugs do, it is worth considering that the improvement in performance the athlete may require is often extremely small and less than the level of significance which may be proved by normal scientific methods. For example, the four minute mile was broken by Sir Roger Bannister in 1954 with a time of 3:59.4 (before electronic timekeeping). In 1981 Sebastian Coe reduced the record to 3:47.33 and in 1985 Steve Cram beat this with a time of 3:46.32. Thus Cram's performance was 5.46 per cent better than Bannister's and 0.4 per cent better than Coe's, averaging less than 0.2 per cent per year. It is hardly surprising therefore, that when a scientific test fails to show a difference between a placebo or a comparator drug in an athletic performance, the sports community fails to consider this as relevant. Lest this comparison be misconstrued, it should not be considered to imply that any of these record breakers have ever misused any drug. Coyle has pointed out that a good training program is the most effective means of improving physical performance and estimates that, in previously sedentary individuals, improvements of 50 per cent are achievable in muscle strength or speed in long-distance running events.[1]

Drug control programmes implemented by most sports governing bodies include the collection and analysis of urine samples from their competitors. Although the great majority of athletes accept the need for controls and indeed wish drug control to succeed, those who are taking banned substances do not wish this use to be detected. In addition, there are too many people who are prepared to sell these substances on the black market and who provide information about their use. The *Underground Steroid Handbook* (USH) is just one such document. Unfortunately, the information contained therein is not always entirely accurate. For example, the USH states that methyltestosterone is undetectable in the steroid tests. This is somewhat surprising since the very first tests for the detection of synthetic anabolic steroid use was based on radioimmunoassays using antibodies raised by Professor R.V. Brooks at St. Thomas' Hospital London. These antibodies were raised to methyltestosterone.

In discussing what the drugs do, it is convenient to consider the various IOC categories, namely stimulants, narcotics, beta-blockers, diuretics and anabolic steroids.

Stimulants

Examples of substances which are included in this category are cocaine, amphetamine, the ephedrines and caffeine.

Cocaine

Although this is one of the most frequently used recreational drugs, apart from anecdotal reports of Peruvians in the Andes chewing leaves of the coca plant, there appear to be no reported studies on the effects of cocaine on athletic performance. The drug acts on catecholaminergic neurons in preventing reuptake of both noradrenaline and dopamine.[2] The physiological effects are similar to those of amphetamine but the mood effects are more profound.

Amphetamines

Smith and Beecher have shown[3] that amphetamines administered two to three hours before a swimming competition produced an increase in time to exhaustion and a small but consistent increase in speed.

Other studies have shown that sprinting speed and muscular strength are not affected by amphetamines.[4,5] Large dose studies on rats[6] (10 to 20 mg/kg) have been shown to be effective in increasing swimming time whereas doses of 1.25 to 5 mg/kg have not produced a significant effect. Treadmill endurance tests have produced similar results.[7]

Ephedrines

Although most people accept the need to control drugs such as amphetamine and cocaine, questions are frequently raised as to whether the restriction of the use of the 'ephedrines' i.e. ephedrine, pseudoephedrine and phenylpropanolamine is necessary. These substances are readily available in most countries in over-the-counter 'cold remedies'.

It is worthwhile to consider the structure-activity relationship of the ephedrines to aid the understanding of their effects as sympathomimetics relative to that of noradrenaline.[8] Substitution at the amino terminal group (figure 6.2) increases β-receptor activity and the smaller the substituent the greater is the selectivity for α-receptor activity. However, N-methylation increases the potency compared to the corresponding primary amine. The presence of hydroxyl groups in the 3 and 4-positions of the aromatic ring results in maximal α- and β-receptor activity. The absence of the polar phenolic hydroxyl groups permits the compound to cross the blood-brain barrier more readily producing greater central activity. Thus, amphetamine, ephedrine and phenylpropanolamine exhibit considerable central nervous system (CNS) activity.

Substitution on the α-carbon atom blocks metabolism by monoamine oxidase of these compounds, allowing them to persist in nerve terminals and hence prolonging the stimulation of the release of noradrenaline from storage sites. An hydroxyl group on the β-carbon atom tends to decrease CNS activity because of reduced lipid solubility. Thus phenylpropanolamine, which is probably the weakest sympathomimetic of the ephedrines, has more marked α- than β-activity because it is a primary amine and because of the hydroxyl group on the β-carbon atom. It has considerable, but often underestimated, CNS activity because of the absence of aromatic substituents. However, this activity is less than that of amphetamine because of the β-substituent which

Figure 6.2 Structure-activity relationship of the ephedrines

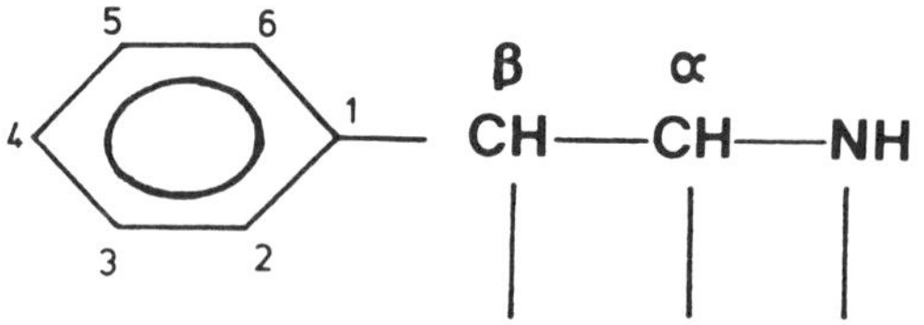

		β	α	
METARAMINOL	3-OH	OH	CH$_3$	CH$_3$
EPHEDRINE		OH	CH$_3$	CH$_3$
AMPHETAMINE		H	CH$_3$	H
PHENYLPROPANOLAMINE		OH	CH$_3$	H

reduces the lipid solubility. Phenylpropanolamine induces hypertension characterised by an increase in cardiac output, peripheral vascular resistance, stroke volume and ejection fraction, and a decrease in heart rate.[9] Even in normal individuals, a typical dose of 75 mg has been shown to have a significant effect and severe hypertension is common after excessive dose and may result in hypertensive encephalopathy, intracerebral haemorrhage, and death.

Caffeine

There is a lack of good dose-response data and the evidence for its central nervous system stimulatory effects is conflicting. However caffeine has been shown to have direct effects on muscle contraction during exercise *in vivo*. Using low frequencies of stimulation increased muscle tension was observed 1 hour after 50 mg caffeine orally but with no apparent difference on endurance time.[10]

Most studies have used a single dose of caffeine ranging from less than 1 to more than 14 mg/kg. Caffeine tolerance may be an explanation for the conflicting results. However, the published data leads one to conclude that doses greater than 400 mg are probably capable of increasing endurance and physical performance. The IOC make it an offence to have a urinary caffeine concentration greater than 12 mg/L (60 µmol/L) and this may be exceeded with a 400 mg dose.

The mechanism for its action is also not certain. Caffeine has been shown to increase calcium permeability which is essential for muscle contraction.[11]

Its action on the CNS may mask fatigue and it has been shown[12] to increase capacity for sustained intellectual effort. Although it may decrease reaction time, fine motor coordination and the ability to judge distance may be impaired. It stimulates the medullary respiratory centres but may produce emesis via the CNS.

Caffeine significantly increases the availability of free fatty acids from fat by lipolysis.[13,14] When available, fatty acids are the primary substrate for aerobic metabolism, thus sparing glycogen. Glucose (produced from glycogen), unlike fatty acids, can be metabolised either aerobically or anaerobically and thus the glycogen spared by the alternative metabolism of fatty acids can be made available at a time when the oxygen supply to the tissues is insufficient for aerobic metabolism.[15] Caffeine has been shown *in vitro* to produce a translocation of intracellular calcium to inhibit phosphodiesterase, thus producing an accumulation of cyclic nucleotides, and also to block the actions of adenosine at adenosine receptors. Amongst its actions, adenosine strongly inhibits hormone-induced lipolysis, reduces the release of noradrenaline from nerve endings and may inhibit the release of excitatory neurotransmitters in the CNS. The concentrations of caffeine required for the translocation of intracellular calcium and the inhibition of phosphodiesterase are greater than are thought to be achieved from a therapeutic dose.[16] Thus, this leaves the blocking of the adenosine receptor as at least one of the most likely routes for caffeine's actions.

Narcotic analgesics

Narcotic analgesics are not perceived by most people as ergogenic drugs. It would seem that the chronic use of narcotics would lead to an impairment of athletic skills.[17] However, the available evidence does not support this assumption. No significant difference has been demonstrated with age-matched controls and addicts in tests of motor strength, rapid alternating movements, eye-hand coordination, visual perception and cognitive skills. Enkephalins and endorphins are endogenous peptides with potent analgesic activity which bind to the sites in the brain to which morphine

Figure 6.3 IOC Medical Commission sports to be tested for beta-blockers

WINTER games	SUMMER games
Biathlon	Archery
Bobsled	Diving and Synchronous swimming
Figure skating—compulsory event	Equestrian
Luge	Fencing
Ski jumping	Gymnastics
	Modern pentathlon—shooting only
	Sailing
	Shooting

and other potent analgesics bind avidly. A correlation between exercise and endorphin activity has been demonstrated.[18] Much of the euphoria experienced by athletes, sometimes known as a 'runner's high' can be explained by a release of some of these endogenous opiates. It has even been suggested [19] that individuals who participate in running may have a type of addiction to these endogenous opiates. On stopping exercising many athletes experience symptoms including anxiety, restlessness, irritability, nervousness, guilt, muscle twitching and sleep disturbances, which may be an 'abstinence syndrome'.

The IOC Medical Commission states that there is evidence indicating that narcotic analgesics have been and are abused in sports. It also justifies their ban on the use of these substances because of the international restrictions affecting the movement of these compounds and comments that their action is in line with the regulations and recommendations of the World Health Organisation regarding narcotics.

Beta-blockers

The IOC Medical Commission has stated that having reviewed the therapeutic indications for the use of beta-blocking drugs it considers that there is now a wide range of effective alternative preparations available in order to control hypertension, cardiac arrhythmias, angina pectoris and migraine. It further states that because of continued misuse of beta-blockers in some sports where physical activity is of no or little importance, it reserves the right to test those sports which it deems appropriate and that these are unlikely to include endurance events. In normal individuals beta-blockers adversely affect both anaerobic endurance and aerobic power as measured by VO_2 max, and time for a 2 km run.[20] Athletes in events such as archery and shooting may gain an advantage from the anxiolytic, bradycardic and anti-tremor effects of the beta-blockers. Table 6.2 indicates those sports which in

September 1987 the IOC Medical Commission decided would be tested for β-blockers at the Olympic Games.

Diuretics

The most obvious reason why athletes may misuse diuretics is to lose body fluid and hence body weight rapidly in order to be able to compete in a lower weight category in those sports where weight is controlled e.g. judo, boxing and rowing. The second and somewhat more obscure reason to misuse diuretics is to reduce the urinary concentration of drugs through rapid diuresis to decrease the likelihood of detection of those drugs in a urine test. There appears to be no study which indicates an enhancement in performance as a result of diuretic use.

Anabolic steroids

This is probably the most notorious of the banned categories of drugs in sport. Although the misuse of anabolic steroids was originally thought to be a problem unique to competitive heavy sports, there is increasing evidence that they are being misused in endurance events and by individuals who do not partake in sports. A survey in the USA revealed that more than 6 per cent of high school males had taken anabolic steroids to make them appear more masculine to their girl friends.

Testosterone is the principal biologically active androgen circulating in the blood of both men and women although women produce about one twentieth of the amount produced by men. The α-reduced form of testosterone is more potent an androgen than testosterone. The reduction predominates in androgen-dependent tissues e.g. the prostate, seminal vesicles and epididymus. Gonadotrophin releasing hormone (GnRH) stimulates the release of luteinising hormone (LH) which in turn stimulates the production of testosterone. Circulating androgens exert a negative feedback on the adenohypophysis and hypothalamus suppressing LH and GnRH release and in this way control the production of the androgens.

Many chemical modifications of testosterone (figure 6.4) have been attempted to alter the anabolic to androgenic ratio (or more muscle per whisker) in order to reduce the virilising androgenic effects or to make the substance orally active. Alkylation at the C-17 position reduces hepatic oxidative metabolism and makes the compound orally active e.g. 17α-methyltestosterone and

Figure 6.4 Chemical modifications of testosterone

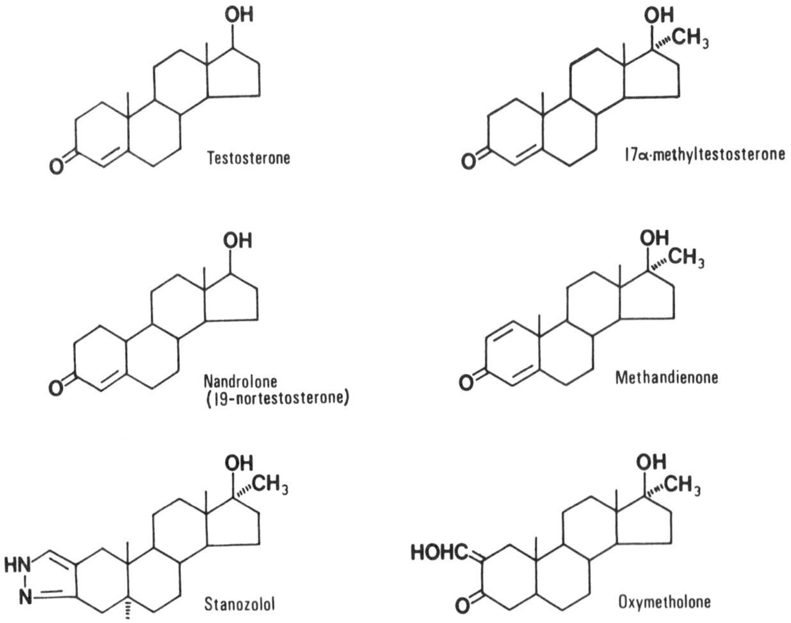

Testosterone

17α-methyltestosterone

Nandrolone
(19-nortestosterone)

Methandienone

Stanozolol

Oxymetholone

methandienone. Removal of the methyl group at C-10 produces nandrolone (19-nortestosterone) which exhibits more anabolic than androgenic activity. Other modifications to increase the anabolic/androgenic ratio are the inclusion of a second double bond in the A-ring, e.g. methandienone, attachment of a pyrazole ring to the A-ring (stanozolol) or a hydroxymethylene group at C-2 (oxymetholone).

Many studies attempting to demonstrate a positive effect of anabolic steroids on sports performance have been conducted over the last 40 years and the reader should consult one of the number of reviews on the subject for more details.[21,22,23] Perhaps the firmest conclusion that may be drawn from these studies is that, if anabolic steroids do have any effect then, their effect is small. Although fluid retention and hence increase in body weight may be one of the first effects observed with anabolic steroid use, some studies have shown that a significant increase in body size and weight can occur not due to fluid retention. These studies observed experienced weight-lifters who continued to train while taking anabolic steroids, and under these circumstances strength was also shown to increase by an amount greater than when not taking anabolic steroids. Generally, the beneficial actions of anabolic steroid are due to anabolic, anti-catabolic and motivational or behavioural effects. Athletes can develop a negative nitrogen balance during excessive training and anabolic steroids may block the effects of the glucocorticoids released from the adrenal cortex in response to the stress of training. Anabolic steroids stimulate erythropoiesis but it is questionable whether the effect is sufficiently significant to enhance performance. On the other hand, erythropoietin produced by recombinant DNA technology is now readily available, and although expensive, is more likely to be misused to increase haemoglobin.

Human chorionic gonadotrophin (HCG) is now being used with anabolic steroids to prevent testicular atrophy because of the androgenic effects of suppressing LH release. HCG mimics the effect of LH and, to a smaller extent follicle stimulating hormone, to help the testes to continue to function normally. The toxicity of anabolic steroids is discussed in a separate chapter by Dr Goldman.

Masking agents and probenecid

The IOC bans pharmacological, chemical and physical methods which alter the integrity and validity of the urine sample collected in a doping control. Specifically, as a pharmacological method, they ban probenecid and related compounds.

Probenecid inhibits the transport of organic acids across epithelial barriers and this is of greatest importance in the renal tubule in which tubular secretion of many drugs and their metabolites is inhibited. However, the excretion of uric acid is increased since its reabsorption in the renal tubule is inhibited by probenecid. Many anabolic steroids are excreted as glucuronic acid conjugates and probenecid can reduce their renal clearance and hence urinary concentration. To be effective, about 2 g of probenecid needs to be taken and probenecid is not difficult for the laboratory to detect in a urine sample.

Growth hormone

No studies to date have shown an increase in strength or endurance in association with human growth hormone (HGH) administration.[24,25] Growth hormone is secreted episodically by the anterior pituitary and has a short half-life of 20 to 30 minutes. Currently produced growth hormone utilises recombinant-DNA technology and although initially it was not an exact duplication (end amino acid was methionine), it now has an identical sequence. Thus it would be extremely difficult to devise a test based on the detection of growth hormone itself to prove that it had been administered in contravention of the rules of sport.

Prior to puberty, excessive HGH gives rise to gigantism. The sufferer tends to die in early adult life from infection, debility or hypopituitarism. After puberty and closure of the long bones, excessive HGH can cause acromegaly with characteristic features such as spade-like hands, lengthened and thickened jaw, coarse and leathery skin, increase in coarse body hair and enlargement of the heart.[26]

HGH release is stimulated by a variety of substances including HGH releasing hormone, noradrenaline, adrenaline (and hence stress), arginine, by insulin (hypoglycaemia), and by sleep. Blood concentrations are reduced by somatostatin and by IGF-1.

The mechanism of action of HGH is far from fully understood. The HGH receptor is widely distributed throughout the body and has been identified on the cell surface membranes of hepatocytes, adipocytes, fibroblasts, lymphocytes and chondrocytes.[27] HGH has been shown, using rat hepatocytes, to cause phosphorylation of certain proteins. This has been shown to be important for the proliferation, differentiation and growth processes and can alter enzymatic activity and cytoskeletal mobility and may modulate events in the nucleus such as gene expression.

Use of bicarbonate: does it enhance performance?

People have used bicarbonate with the aim of increasing the buffering capacity of blood and hence to counteract the buildup of lactic acid resulting from anaerobic glycolysis which would inhibit glycolysis and cause fatigue. Provided that the exercise is not primarily aerobic and the dose is adequate, bicarbonate has been shown to enhance exercise time to exhaustion.[28] Large amounts are required (more than 300 mg/kg) and this will cause diarrhoea in most subjects. Chronic administration can cause hypercalcaemia and alkalosis which can cause changes in electrolyte balance and respiration, potentially with serious consequences.

Bicarbonate has previously been used to alkalinise the urine in order to increase the reabsorption of basic drugs in the renal tubes and hence to reduce the urinary excretion and hence concentration of these substances. However, modern analytical methods are sufficiently sensitive to make this technique ineffective in evading detection. At the present time, the use of bicarbonate is not normally controlled in sport although urinary pH is sometimes checked at the time of sample collection.

Clenbuterol

Clenbuterol is a β-selective adrenergic agonist which has been shown to stimulate the deposition of body protein and inhibit that of body fat in animals.[29] It has a very small therapeutic dose in man (10 to 40 µg day) and a relatively long half-life of about 30 hours. Its anabolic and anti-lipogenic actions are mechanistically distinct and there is growing concern that it is being misused in sport for its anabolic properties.

Can We Detect the Drugs? Are Our Methods Sensitive Enough?

Some indication of what maybe detected is apparent by inspection of the findings of IOC accredited laboratories (figure 6.5). These figures should not be considered as representative of the scale of misuse. Most of the samples have been collected at competitions and may be further biased by the sampling protocol which may, for example, be to sample the first, second and third for one event. Neither should these figures be used to determine the relative abuse of the different substances. The detectability of the substance depends not only on the analytical technique employed but also on the elimination profile of the particular substance, which may be represented by the half-life, and by its formulation, e.g. cocaine has a plasma half-life of about 1 hour, caffeine has a plasma half-life of about 3.5 hours whereas that of an oily injection of a nandrolone ester will be measured in days.

The IOC Medical Commission has stated that it wishes to control those drugs which may be harmful when misused and to do this with the minimum interference to the normal therapeutic use of drugs. Far more drugs are permitted than are banned. This is very different from the sport of horseracing where nearly everything that is not a normal nutrient is banned.

The number of samples collected worldwide has increased over the last few years but even in 1989 was only about 52 000, representing only a very small proportion of athletes in top-level sport. Approximately 2 per cent of the samples analysed have been found to contain one or more substances from the banned classes. The commonest group have been the anabolic steroids with nandrolone being the commonest substance in that group and testosterone the

Figure 6.5 IOC-accredited laboratories: statistics

Summary of samples analysed 1986 to 1989

Year	Number of samples	Number of negative samples	Number of analytically positive A-samples	%	Labs
1986	32 982	32 359	623	1.89	18
1987	37 882	37 028	854	2.25	21
1988	47 069	45 916	1 153	2.45	20
1989	52 371	51 165	1 206	2.30	20

Summary of identified substances

IOC category	1989	%	1988	%	1987	%	1986	%
A. Stimulants	508	40.4	420	31.0	300	31.9	177	26.3
B. Narcotics	76	6.1	58	4.3	55	5.8	23	3.4
C. Anabolic Steroids	611	48.6	791	58.5	521	55.4	439	65.3
D. Beta-blockers	6	0.5	8	0.6	32	3.4	31	4.6
E. Diuretics	45	3.6	57	4.2	9	1.0	2	0.3
Masking agents	10	0.8	19	1.4	24	2.6		
TOTAL	1256		1353		941		672	

N.B. Some samples contain more than one substance from banned classes.

IOC category	COMMONEST FINDING	YEAR		
		1987	1988	1989
Stimulants	Ephedrines	215	297	374
Narcotics	Codeine	26	35	34
Anabolic Steroids	Nandrolone	262	304	224
Beta-blockers	Propranolol	19	7	3
Diuretics	Frusemide	8	35	15
Masking agents	Probenecid	1–1	19	10

second most common. The ephedrines are the most frequently found substances in the stimulant category. Note that betà-blockers are controlled only in certain sports and hence the figures relating to their finding depend on whether those sports have been tested. For further details, see Appendix 6.1

Conclusion

This chapter illustrates the variety of substances which have been used in sport in an attempt to enhance performance. The athlete does not appear to be deterred by any lack of scientific evidence that the substance is efficacious, nor by the documented risk of potentially hazardous side-effects. The whole area is dynamic, advancing as science advances. There is a definite need to improve our understanding of whether and how the substances work and, although many are detectable by current analytical methods, new techniques are needed to meet and to anticipate the new challenges. Ultimately, however, what is use and what represents misuse is a moral question which all in society and sport must answer.

Appendix 6.1

Examples and explanations of IOC drug bans and restrictions

I. DOPING CLASSES

A. Stimulants

amfepramone
amfetaminil
amiphenazole
amphetamine
benzphetamine
caffeine*
cathine
chlorphentermine
clobenzorex
clorprenaline
cocaine
cropropamide (component
of Micoren)
crotethamide (component
of Microren)
dimetamfetamine
ephedrine
etafedrine
ethamivan
etilamfetamine

fencamfamin
fenetylline
fenproporex
furfenorex
mefenorex
methamphetamine
methoxyphenamine
methylephedrine
methylphenidate
morazone
nikethamide
pemoline
pentetrazol
phendimetrazine
phenmetrazine
phentermine
phenylpropanolamine
pipradol
prolintane

* For caffeine the definition of a positive depends upon the following: if the concentration in urine exceeds 12 micrograms/ml.

propylhexedrine   strychnine
pyrovalerone
                          and related compounds

Stimulants comprise various types of drugs which increase alertness, reduce fatigue and may increase competitiveness and hostil-
ity. Their use can also produce loss of judgement, which may lead
to accidents to others in some sports. Amphetamine and related
compounds have the most notorious reputation in producing problems in sport. Some deaths of sportsmen have resulted when
normal doses have been used under conditions of maximum physical activity. There is no medical justification for the use of stimulants. One group of stimulants is the sympathomimetic amines of
which ephedrine is an example. In high doses, this type of compound produces mental stimulation and increased blood flow.
Adverse effects include elevated blood pressure and headache,
increased and irregular heart beat, anxiety and tremor. In lower
doses, they e.g. ephedrine, pseudoephedrine, phenylpropanolamine, norpseudoephedrine, are often present in cold and hay
fever preparations which can be purchased in pharmacies and
sometimes from other retail outlets without the need of a medical
prescription.

*THUS NO PRODUCT FOR USE IN COLDS, FLU OR HAY
FEVER PURCHASED BY A COMPETITOR OR GIVEN TO
HIM/HER SHOULD BE USED WITHOUT FIRST CHECKING
WITH A DOCTOR OR PHARMACIST THAT THE PRODUCT
DOES NOT CONTAIN A DRUG OF THE BANNED
STIMULANTS CLASS.*

Beta2 agonists

The choice of medication in the treatment of asthma and respiratory ailments has posed many problems. Some years ago,
ephedrine and related substances were administered quite frequently. However, these substances are prohibited because they are
classed in the category of 'sympathomimetic amines' and therefore
considered as stimulants.
    The use of only the following beta2 agonists is permitted in the
aerosol form: bitolterol, orciprenaline, rimiterol, salbutamol,
terbutaline.

B. *Narcotic analgesics*

alphaprodine	ethoheptazine
anileridine	ethylmorphine
buprenorphine	levorphanol
codeine	methadone
dextromoramide	morphine
dextropropoxyphen	nalbuphine
diamorphine (heroin)	pentazocine
dihydrocodeine	pethidine
dipipanone	phenazocine
	trimeperidine

and related compounds

The drugs belonging to this class, which are represented by morphine and its chemical and pharmacological analogues, act fairly specifically as analgesics for the management of moderate to severe pain. This description, however, by no means implies that their clinical effect is limited to the relief of trivial disabilities. Most of these drugs have major side effects, including dose-related respiratory depression, and carry a high risk of physical and psychological dependence. There exists evidence indicating that narcotic analgesics have been and are abused in sports, and therefore the IOC Medical Commission has issued and maintained a ban on their use during the Olympic Games. The ban is also justified by international restrictions affecting the movement of these compounds and is in line with the regulations and recommendations of the World Health Organisation regarding narcotics.

Furthermore, it is felt that the treatment of slight to moderate pain can be effective using drugs—other than the narcotics—which have analgesic, anti-inflammatory and antipyretic actions. Such alternatives, which have been successfully used for the treatment of sports injuries, include anthranilic acid derivatives (such as mefenamic acid, Floctafenine, Glafenine etc.), phenylalkanoic acid derivatives (such as Diclofenac, Ibuprofen, Ketoprofen, Naproxen etc.) and compounds such as Indomethacin and Sulindac. The Medical Commission also reminds athletes and team doctors that aspirin and its newer derivatives (such as Diflunisal) are not banned but cautions against some pharmaceutical preparations where aspirin is often associated to a banned drug such as codeine. The same precautions hold for cough and cold preparations which often contain drugs of the banned classes.

DEXTROMETHORPHAN AND PHOLCODINE ARE NOT
BANNED AND MAY BE USED AS ANTI-TUSSIVES.
DIPHENOXYLATE IS ALSO PERMITTED.

C. *Anabolic steroids*

bolasterone	methyltetosterone
boldenone	nandrolone
clostebol	norethandrolone
dehydrochlormethyltestosterone	oxandrolone
fluoxymesterone	oxymesterone
mesterolone	oxymetholone
metandienone	stanozolol
metenolone	testosterone*

and related compounds

This class of drugs includes chemicals which are related in structure and activity to the male hormone testosterone, which is also included in this banned class. They have been misused in sport, not only to attempt to increase muscle bulk, strength and power when used with increased food intake, but also in lower doses and normal food intake to attempt to improve competitiveness.

Their use in teenagers who have not fully developed can result in stunting growth by affecting growth at the ends of the long bones. Their use can produce psychological changes, liver damage and adversely affect the cardiovascular system. In males, their use can reduce testicular size and sperm production; in females, their use can produce masculinisation, acne, development of male pattern hair growth and suppression of ovarian function and menstruation.

D. *Beta-blockers*

acebutolol	nadolol
alprenolol	oxprenolol
atenolol	propranolol
labetalol	sotalol
metoprolol	

and related compounds

The IOC Medical Commission has reviewed the therapeutic indications for the use of betà-blocking drugs and noted that there is

---

* Testosterone: the definition of a positive depends upon the following—the administration of testosterone or the use of any other manipulation having the result of increasing the ratio in urine of testosterone/epitestosterone to above 6.

now a wide range of effective alternative preparations available in order to control hypertension, cardiac arrhythmias, angina pectoris and migraine. Due to the continued misuse of beta-blockers in some sports where physical activity is of no or little importance, the IOC Medical Commission reserves the right to test those sports which it deems appropriate. These are unlikely to include endurance events which necessitate substrates in which beta-blockers would severely decrease performance capacity.

E. *Diuretics*

acetazolamide	diclofenamide
amiloride	ethacrynic acid
bendroflumethiazide	furosemide
benzthiazide	hydrochlorothiazide
bumetanide	mersalyl
canrenone	spironolactone
chlormerodrin	triamterene
chlortalidone	

and related compounds

Diuretics have important therapeutic indications for the elimination of fluids from the tissues in certain pathological conditions. However, strict medical control is required.

Diuretics are sometimes misused by competitors for two main reasons, namely: to reduce weight quickly in sports where weight categories are involved and to reduce the concentration of drugs in urine by producing a more rapid excretion of urine to attempt to minimise detection of drug misuse. Rapid reduction of weight in sport cannot be justified medically. Health risks are involved in such misuse because of serious side-effects which might occur.

Furthermore, deliberate attempts to reduce weight artificially in order to compete in lower weight classes or to dilute urine constitute clear manipulations which are unacceptable on ethical grounds. Therefore, the IOC Medical Commission has decided to include diuretics on its list of banned classes of drugs.

FOR SPORTS INVOLVING WEIGHT CLASSES, THE IOC MEDICAL COMMISSION RESERVES THE RIGHT TO OBTAIN URINE SAMPLES FROM THE COMPETITOR AT THE TIME OF THE WEIGH-IN.

F. *Peptide hormones and analogues*

Chorionic gonadotrophin (HCG, human chorionic gonadotrophin.)
It is well known that the administration to males of human chorionic gonadotrophin (HCG) and other compounds with related activity leads to an increased rate of production of endogenous androgenic steroids and is considered equivalent to the exogenous administration of testosterone.

Corticotrophin (ACTH).
Corticotrophin has been misused to increase the blood levels of endogenous corticosteroids notably to obtain the euphoric effect of corticosteroids. The application of corticotrophin is considered to be equivalent to the oral, intramuscular or intravenous application of corticosteroids. (See Section III. D).

Growth hormone (HGH, somatotrophin).
The misuse of growth hormone in sport is deemed to be unethical and dangerous because of various adverse effects, for example, allergic reactions, diabetogenic effects, and acromegaly when applied in high doses.

ALL THE RESPECTIVE RELEASING FACTORS OF THE ABOVE-MENTIONED SUBSTANCES ARE ALSO BANNED.

Erythropoietin (EPO).
Is the glucoprotein hormone produced in the human kidney which regulates, apparently by a feed-back mechanism, the rate of synthesis of erythrocytes.

II. *METHODS*

A. *Blood doping*

Blood transfusion is the intravenous administration of red blood cells or related blood products that contain red blood cells. Such products can be obtained from blood drawn from the same (autologous) or from a different (non-autologous) individual. The most common indications for red blood cell transfusion in conventional medical practice are acute blood loss and severe anaemia.

Blood doping is the administration of blood or related red blood products to an athlete other than for legitimate medical treatment. This procedure may be preceded by withdrawal of blood from the athlete who continues to train in this blood depleted state.

These procedures contravene the ethics of medicine and of sport. There are also risks involved in the transfusion of blood and related blood products. These include the development of allergic reactions (rash, fever etc.) and acute haemolytic reaction with kidney damage if incorrectly typed blood is used, as well as delayed transfusion reaction resulting in fever and jaundice, transmission of infectious diseases (viral hepatitis and AIDS), overload of the circulation and metabolic shock.

Therefore, the practice of blood doping in sport is banned by the IOC Medical Commission.

The IOC Medical Commission bans erythropoietin as a method of doping (see section 1.F).

B. *Pharmacological, chemical and physical manipulation*

The IOC Medical Commission bans the use of substances and of methods which alter the integrity and validity of urine samples used in doping controls. Examples of banned methods are catheterisation, urine substitution and/or tampering, inhibition of renal excretion e.g. by probenecid and related compounds.

III. *CLASSES OF DRUGS SUBJECT TO CERTAIN RESTRICTIONS*

A. *Alcohol*

Alcohol is not prohibited. However, breath or blood alcohol levels may be determined at the request of an international federation.

B. *Marijuana*

Marijuana is not prohibited. However, tests may be carried out at the request of an international federation.

C. *Local Anaesthetics*

Injectable local anaesthetics are permitted under the following conditions:
• that procaine, xylocaine, carbocaine etc. are used but not cocaine
• only local or intra-articular injections maybe administered
• only when medically justified (i.e. the details including diagnosis, dose and route of administration must be submitted immediately in writing to the IOC Medical Commission)

D. *Corticosteroids*

The naturally occurring and synthetic corticosteroids are mainly used as anti-inflammatory drugs which also relieve pain. They influence circulating concentrations of natural corticosteroids in the body. They produce euphoria and side-effects such that their medical use, except when used topically, requires medical control. Since 1975, the IOC Medical Commission has attempted to restrict their use during the Olympic Games by requiring a declaration by the team doctors, because it was known that corticosteroids were being used non-therapeutically by the oral, intramuscular and even the intravenous route in some sports. However, the problem was not solved by these restrictions and therefore stronger measures designed not to interfere with the appropriate medical use of these compounds became necessary.

The use of corticosteroids is banned except for topical use (aural, ophthalmological and dermatological), inhalational therapy (asthma, allergic rhinitis) and local or intra-articular injections.

ANY TEAM DOCTOR WISHING TO ADMINISTER CORTICOSTEROIDS INTRA-ARTICULARLY OR LOCALLY TO A COMPETITOR MUST GIVE WRITTEN NOTIFICATION TO THE IOC MEDICAL COMMISSION.

7 The need for steroids in modern athletism
Saxon White

The general thrust of this book discusses the ancient conundrum of whether athletes should take drugs, why they do take them, and what detrimental effects on health do they risk in the pursuit of a winning edge. In this context the act of taking performance-boosting aids raises other issues. What is fair and unfair play? If an athlete has an inherent health defect, what actions are permissible to allow him/her to compete from an equal psychological and physiological base? Good examples of the latter in modern sport are the needs of asthmatic and diabetic athletes, who are allowed to take drugs to compete.

While society in general continues to try to work its way through the problem, the physiologist has an increasing anxiety, born out of his/her insight into the needs of the athlete, that the natural effects of modern training might actually *disadvantage* the athlete physiologically when all expectations are to the contrary. Need we be reminded of the time, artistically put to us in the film *Chariots of Fire*, when special training schedules and advice were looked upon with disdain. Be that as it may, it will be argued in this chapter that training in itself may certainly hinder the athlete of modern times in such a way that drugs are a *requirement* to keep the athlete fit.

The current discussions in our Human Performance Laboratory of the Hunter Academy of Sport focus on the female, and I believe one of the more fascinating and hidden outcomes of the finding that high-level training *disadvantages* the female is that women themselves will widen the coming debate about the need for drugs to keep the female Olympic athlete healthy, to an insistence that men and women compete against each other. For this reason the IOC, and indeed other unrelated sporting bodies, will need to devise far reaching policies concerning *the need for drugs* in order to cope with the profound effects of modern training methods on human physiology. In 1991 these considerations are quite new, and moreover, they may be sex-specific.

In 1974 the question was raised concerning the value of fat (women's secret weapon[1]) as a sex-related advantageous source of energy for running long distance events including the marathon. Such a theory foreshadowed the running of the first women's marathon in Los Angeles in 1984. Dr Wendy Brown in my laboratory coupled this question with the work of Gorsky,[2] who showed at least in the endurance-swimming rat that oestrogen enhanced carbohydrate parsimony thereby causing the rat to use a greater proportion of fat as its energy source. Could oestrogen drive metabolism in the human female and thereby provide for a better mix of substrate during endurance performance to ease her past that critical point towards the end of the marathon where her limited carbohydrate stores might otherwise become exhausted?

Athletes call the phenomenon of physical exhaustion at this time 'hitting the wall', and it has been suggested that this is a characteristic of male runners rather than women. We perceived then that if the theory that women burn relatively more fat then men were true there would be a cost, in that burning a greater proportion of fat requires greater oxygen needs. This would place a greater if small demand (4 to 10 per cent) in women on factors responsble for oxygen transport e.g. on the heart, and this could paradoxically *blunt* a winning edge. Nevertheless, any advantage the male might gain in greater capacities for energy (glycogen) storage due to his greater testosterone[3] production prior to the race, would be offset by the disadvantage of not having oestrogen to spin out his carbohydrate stores over the two plus hours of marathon running.

We tested the postulate of a substrate-usage advantage in the female due to a unique oestrogen/fat link by observing the commencing rate, and rate of change, of substrate utilisation (using the indirect measure of respiratory exchange ratio) in trained and untrained men and women over a two-hour endurance effort. It turned out that women do appear to utilise a greater background proportion of fat than men at the commencement of the endurance effort, and there is a suggestion that this effect is more prominent in those that exercise *least* i.e. untrained women! However, the rate of change toward greater fat utilisation as the endurance effort proceeded is exactly the same in men and women whether trained or untrained. Only in a separate group of the most highly trained males, who preferentially burned carbohydrate as they commenced, did we detect a more rapid rate of carbohydrate utilisation over the two hour period. But in general we thought the theory was not substantiated, unless of course the males were producing significant oestradiol themselves.

To our surprise, we found that oestrogen levels in the trained male athlete, and in untrained men, were as high during exercise as in the early follicular and late luteal phases of the menstrual cycle of the women. Several conclusions were inevitable. These were that if the Gorsky data provided insight into how substrate utilisation is driven by oestrogen in the female during endurance exercise, then it was probably also true of the male. Moreover taking into account the characteristically different serum oestrogen/testosterone concentration ratio between the sexes, our data suggested the Gorsky effect during endurance exercise was not concentration-dependent i.e. the effect would occur irrespective of low, or high, concentrations of the hormone.

Nothing daunted, this second postulate was examined further in studies[4] on prepubertal (according to rigid scientific criteria) children of the Nelson Bay area of the Hunter Region. Untrained boys and girls of average age 10 years carried out an endurance exercise protocol over 90 minutes at 60 per cent of their predetermined maximal oxygen uptake; respiratory exchange ratio was again used as an indirect index of their substrate utilisation. As expected, their sex hormone concentrations were very low at rest, and did not change appreciably during exercise, but other hormones such as growth hormone, cortisol, androstenedione and in the girls, 17-hydroxyprogesterone, did rise. Nevertheless *commencing* substrate utilisation between the sexes reflected the pattern of difference previously noted between *adult* men and women, where there is a greater proportion of background fat utilisation in the females compared to the males. Likewise, *during* endurance exercise, the slow *rate of fall* in carbohydrate and rise in fat utilisation over 90 minutes is identical to that seen in adults.

These data confirm the female propensity to burn a greater proportion of fat *at rest and during exercise* compared to the male and that, if the pattern is dependent on the female hormone, then it is concentration independent. An alternative hypothesis is that the effect may not be specific to oestrogen alone, but rather to a profile of hormones with overlapping effects on metabolism, for example, oestrogen, growth hormone, progesterone and cortisone. Nevertheless, it follows that the differences between men and women when commencing exercise reflect the oestrogen/testosterone concentration ratio, and that the change in carbohydrate/fat utilisation during endurance exercise reflects the rise in concentration of the mix of sex and other hormones. It may also be predicted that the carbohydrate/fat metabolism of postmenopausal women and their male counterparts during endurance events would follow a similar pattern. This postulate remains untested.

The systematic lower set point of substrate utilisation in favour of greater fat utilisation in the female, irrespective of training and pubertal status also suggests that she is at any instant burning a greater proportion of fat than the male irrespective of the size of her carbohydrate store. Because the male uses a greater proportion of carbohydrate for energy production at rest and during exercise, it follows he would certainly be more vulnerable in the marathon than his female counterpart.

Changes in body physiology brought about by repetitive athletic training

Physiologists were first alerted to the impact of physical activity on body control systems by the phenomenon of irregular occurrence, and even complete cessation, of the menstrual cycle in the female athlete. At first a curiosity, it attracted greater attention in modern times *pari passu* with the emancipation of women socially and as athletes. Indeed, over the past 20 years the interest of the physiologist and medical practitioner in modern athleticism has paralleled the intensity of training programs and the realisation that the altered menstrual cycle reflected the tip of a massive iceberg of altered control systems, and not just those related to the menstrual cycle. For example, in 1987 we linked a theory of cause of the irregular menstrual cycle to a similar mechanism for lowering resting arterial pressure by exercise.[5]

It is now apparent that some of the outcome phenomena of training we observe are primary, and others are secondary to the primary disturbance. Not only is this theory plausible, but it has a universal application in explaining many other symptoms and signs which have recently become apparent as real health problems in women *and men* subjected to the intense training regimens of the modern athlete. Moreover it predicts the appearance of future problems, their mechanism and management.

As mentioned above, in untrained and trained women and men in the reproductive age group exercise evokes a rise in serum oestrogen concentration. It has been suggested that the much greater frequency of exercise training bouts and rises in hormone

Figure 7.1 Schematic representation of possible sex hormone suppressing mechanisms in male and female athletes

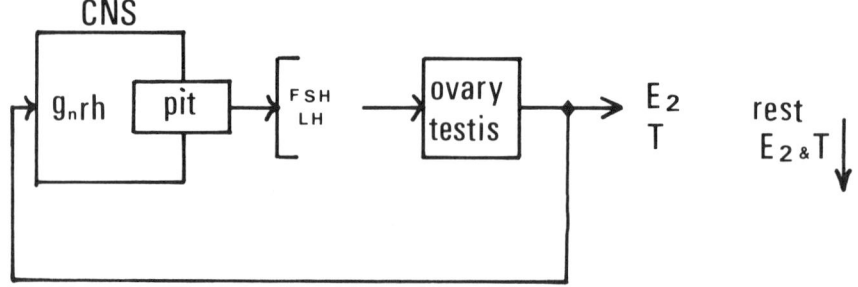

Note: One theory to explain why women and men develop depressed levels of sex hormones (E_2 = oestrogen; T = testosterone) due to extensive training over many months/years concerns the effects of repetitive rises of these hormones provoked by repetitive training and competition bouts of exercise. The more frequent-than-usual rises in these hormones 'switch-off' brain (CNS: central nervous system) hormones (GnRH: gonadotropin releasing hormone) responsible for stimulating the release of pituitary (pit) follicle-stimulating hormone (FSH) and luteinising hormone (LH) which normally act on the ovary and testis, the production sites of oestrogen and testosterone, respectively. The lack of stimulation results in low *resting* levels of the sex hormones and in the possibility of fertility changes in women and men.

levels over unit time in the female athlete, cause feedback 'inhibition', in line with the accepted physiological theory, of those brain regions and mechanisms (in the hypothalamic and pituitary organs) responsible for driving the normal cycle of hormones responsible for menstruation. A similar theory is advanced for men, where the repetitive exercise-provoked rise in testosterone (the source of oestrogen in men following conversion of testosterone by the aromatase enzyme in peripheral tissues) indirectly 'switches off' testosterone production in the testes between exercise bouts, by inhibiting the hormones normally released from the brain to stimulate the testes.

The sensitivity of this mechanism for depressing the menstrual cycle appears to vary considerably between women (some get it, and some do not) and indeed between the training regimens which characterise different sports e.g. the effect may be less prominent in swimming than in running, gymnastics and ballet. We are also aware that the effects go beyond a simple alteration of the physiological behaviour of the athlete's body, and can become incapacitating. A simplified schematic representation of the oestrogen and blood pressure suppression mechanisms is shown in figures 7.1 and 7.2.

Figure 7.2 Schematic representation of possible arterial pressure-reducing mechanisms in athletes

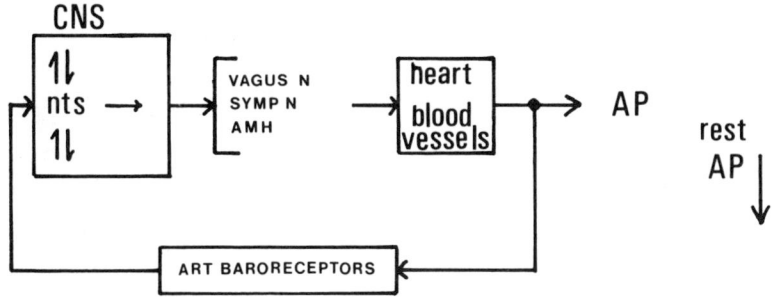

Note: Another example of how repetitive exercise bouts in training regimes may affect control systems in the athlete, this time with respect to arterial pressure (AP). Exercise-induced bouts of increased AP stimulate the blood pressure receptors (art baroreceptors), which in turn affect brain (CNS: central nervous system) mechanisms (nts: nucleus tractus solitarius and associated pathways) so that *at rest*, the blood pressure control mechanisms (vagus and sympathetic nerves, and adrenal medullary hormones) behave as though the blood pressure is persistently elevated. This parallels the behaviour of the pituitary hormones FSH and LH, which behave as though oestrogen and testosterone in women and men are persistently elevated. At rest, therefore, there is lowered heart rate (vagal effect) and withdrawal of sympathetic nerve and adrenal medullary hormone activity, resulting in lowered arterial pressure.

While the effects of exercise on both the menstrual cycle and blood pressure are reversible e.g. the menstrual cycle will return to normal in runners and ballet dancers on cessation of training, sophisticated testing suggests that the reproductive control system in question can 'reset' permanently. In 1990 much research needs to be done to help us understand the details in terms of underlying cause of these phenomena. For example, in female runners in the reproductive age group, there are persistently low serum levels of the hormones oestrogen and prolactin, and altered thyroid function leading to sub-clinical hypothyroidism. Also, the brain hormones responsible for stimulating ovarian hormone release show reduced responses to provocative tests. In male distance runners, there is reduced serum testosterone and prolactin levels, and in the extreme, evidence of lowered sperm counts,[6] showing that the effects of training on the reproductive system are not specific to the female.

But just to show how sensitive these hormonal control systems may be, we investigated in 1989 the prevalence of menstrual problems in teenage (15-year-old) ballet dancers[7] (illustration) and their matched school-friend controls in the Hunter Region of New South

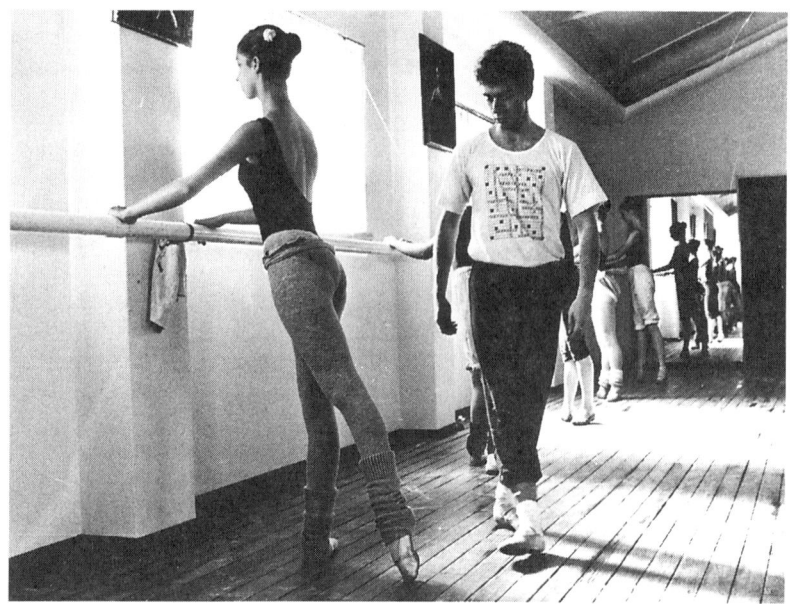

A 15-year-old ballerina at the barre in the Robyn Turner Ballet School, Newcastle, Australia. These teenagers have lower serum oestrogen and higher serum testosterone levels at rest and during exercise compared to matched controls, and this endocrine disturbance probably accounts for their altered menstrual cycle.

Wales. We found a 71 per cent prevalence (compared to 19 per cent in the controls) even though the dancers showed no detectable difference from their friends in aerobic fitness, diet, skin fold thickness or size (weight and height). The dancers however showed significantly higher testosterone and lower serum oestrogen concentrations than their non-dancing friends, although the values were within the normal range for 15-year-olds. The dancers also had a higher serum concentration of follicle stimulating hormone. These findings suggest that the first effects of female athleticism are transitional, and focus on the peripheral conversion of testosterone to oestrogen perhaps in the ovary. But with the more intense training of professional ballet, or track, the hormone profile and control system modifications change to the more central, adult 'derangement'. Work is continuing on these fascinating areas of athlete hormone controls.

Exercise programs also lower blood pressure, both in the controlled laboratory environment,[8] and in community fitness centres,[9] and reset downwards the activity of the sympathetic nervous system. The mechanisms of all these effects are postulated to result from frequent repetitive rises in arterial pressure and heart rate— and in a variety of hormones e.g. adrenal medullary hormones, the sex hormones, growth hormone, thyroid hormone and so on—as a consequence of repetitive athletic training. If this is carried out over many years, it has been speculated that in its most gross form those most sensitive will show some permanency of effect manifest in amenorrhoea (complete loss of the menstrual cycle), problems of reproduction, hypotension and hypothyroidism and a greater like-lihood of incapacitating syndromes such as exercise-induced asthma, and osteoporosis with associated stress fractures.

One example of the gathering storm for the modern female athlete is the puzzle of osteoporosis. Where oestrogen in low con-centrations may play a permissive role rather than a concentration-dependent role in driving fat metabolism, its role in calcium metabolism may be more quantitative. In 1984[10] Cann, using computerised tomography, found bony decalcification in spinal vertebral bone in young adult women with ovarian 'failure' syn-dromes, and this has been followed by similar findings in women with anorexia nervosa and running-induced menstrual problems. Trabecular bone densities in amenorrhoeic runners are in the aver-age range of women aged 50 years, and appear to be associated with increased risk of stress fractures. While radial bone density appears protected trabecular bone, e.g. in vertebra, is not, but the latter will recover vertebral density by some 6.2 per cent in four-teen months following the return of the menstrual cycle with the lessening of training exercise.

Oestrogen levels can be extraordinarily low in the female athlete and in postmenopausal women, in whom stress fractures are rela-tively common. With the recent demonstration of oestrogen recep-tors in bone to account for this phenomenon, oestrogen is considered to play a pivotal role in the dynamic maintenance of the collagen-calcium framework of bone. A fall in oestrogen con-centration results in matrix breakdown, calcium release into body fluids and fractures in those resorptive sites most at risk to sheer stress and compression forces e.g. the vertebral bodies, and at sites in the lower limbs.

But the fall in oestradiol is physiologically coupled with a reduction in the hormone calcitonin, which normally *prevents* bone resorption. The tendency for serum calcium to rise also results in secondary inhibition of parathormone release, a reduction in calciferol manufacture in the kidney, and decreased calcium reabsorption from the intestine. The inhibition of parathormone highlights the presence of helpful mechanisms *restraining* osteoporosis. Thus, should repetitive exercise cause any lowering of concentrations of hormones such as parathormone, thyroid hormone, or cortisol, bony resorption would be *restrained*. Since current evidence suggests that hormones such as parathormone, thyroid hormone and cortisol in the female athlete at rest are indeed normal, or lowered, it is clear why *the fall in oestrogen production in the repetitively trained adult female is seen as the key event for osteoporosis*. The fact that prepubertal children and men are less prone to osteoporosis also marks clearly the supportive role for other hormones, such as growth hormone (which exerts a powerful positive effect on intestinal absorption of calcium) and calcitonin (which enhances bone formation).

With this in mind, primary reduction in resting oestrogen concentration may be perceived to precipitate a kind of downward reset of bone metabolism, which is restrained in part by the positive effects of repetitive exercise stress on bony radial density, and in part by the fall in other hormones which only in excess, cause negative calcium balance. It is notable that other steroid hormones including cortisone are in this class, so that any addition of exogenous steroid hormones such as cortisone to the female training package may *enhance* the lowered oestrogen effects on bone, and exacerbate osteoporosis. There are anecdotal reports of cortisone abuse in Australian athletes in 1991, mainly for their enhancement of a feeling of 'well-being' during tough training schedules.

The idea that modern, high-level intensive training regimes have untoward effects on the resting, and response, profile of control systems immediately raises questions of medical management. Medical management initiatives have been raised by the athlete, the coach, administrators and within the medical profession. Most athletes however including dancers, male and female, are locked into financially rewarding career development patterns that demand a continuance of training. They cannot simply stop training, a process we know will usually (but not always) reverse the resetting of physiological control systems and result in a return to a normal physiological state.

As this is written, we are seeing an increasing number of articles[11] advising on oestrogen hormone regimes for women who are involved in high-level physical activity. The articles advise on regimes which will restrain and even improve bone mineralisation in the female in training. What will our club, national, and Olympic organisations think about this? Is this a form of *steroid taking that will protect the athlete*? And is this a form a therapy that will correct an endogenous defect and return the athlete to competing on an equal footing (as in asthma)? Or is this a form of therapy that will provide the athlete with an *illegal* advantage? On scientific grounds she will certainly be better off than a female counter-part who is equally trained but *not* taking exogenous oestrogen, because she will have less bony demineralisation, less susceptibility to fractures, and with careful manipulation of the hormone, a menstrual cycle tailored to fit her training and racing schedule. Moreover, she will ensure that her metabolism, at least in endurance events, is superior to men in relation to the use of fat and carbohydrate as an energy source. She will not be subject to 'hitting the wall'.

All the above considerations make many a scientist uneasy about the lack of *appropriate* policy with respect to drugs and athletic performance. There is little doubt that the only way out of these problems is to work through them as a community of athletes, coaches, scientists, philosophers and administrators. But once women understand that their inherent sex hormone makeup may provide an advantage over men, at least in endurance events, the female community will most certainly demand an increasing number of competitive events in which the sexes compete against each other. And then the sociological fat will be in the fire.

8 The doping problem in sport: from drugs to genetic engineering
Ronald Laura

In this chapter I shall be concerned to argue that the central problem confronting the world of sport today is *not* the elimination of the vast array of drugs used to enhance sporting performance. As important and pressing as this issue is, the problem of drugs in sport reflects in the final analysis only a symptom of a much deeper problem. The deeper problem involves the loss or failure of a philosophy of sport which motivates 'play' for its own sake—for the 'love of the game', if you like—and which sees sporting interaction as an activity which serves to enhance human integrity rather than just human performance. As long as the goal of sporting games presupposes that winning is in itself an ultimate value, the temptation will be to forsake *the value of being the best that one can be* in favour of simply being better than one's competitors.

To be determined—indeed, driven—to be better than one's competitors has become an obscene obsession within sport. It is obscene because the values it fosters pressure athletes to be not just the best they can be but paradoxically, to be even better than they can be; to extend, that is to say, one's sporting capabilities through the use of exogenous performance-boosting agents, beyond the ambit of what one is capable of providing oneself. So long as the goal of sporting competition is dominated by interests independent of sport, such as the financial gains to be made from sport, athletes will do whatever they must to win. This being so, it is no surprise that athletes are willing to use their own bodies, and in certain sports the bodies of their competitors, as little more than the means to an end. On the other hand, the goal of being better than one's competitors may also on some occasions be insufficient to inspire an athlete to strive to be the best that he or she can be. We have all perhaps seen—at some time or other—an athlete who won without 'really trying', without having given his or her best effort, and in a bizarre sense we have all felt cheated. The reason we feel cheated—despite the triumph—is that we have been deprived of the experience of bearing witness to the realisation of human potential; an experience we still value, though all too dimly on the field of play. What we experience instead is an event in which the *best* performance the athlete could have given on the day is substituted for a *winning* performance. The two are not one and the same, nor do they have the same value.

Inasmuch as the value of sport has become progressively focused upon the value of winning, my argument is that the eradication of drugs in sport would serve as no more than a cosmetic resolution to a fundamental problem of value and philosophy in sport. By treating the symptom of a disease without attending to its aetiology, we allow the disease to reappear in due course and manifest in a new and undoubtedly equally pernicious form. In regard to the drug problem in sport, we would in the end simply be substituting one form of performance-boosting perversion for another.

Given that we were successful in our campaign to eradicate drugs from sport, it would in any case be just a matter of time before the technology available to us would be used to confer an advantage upon those athletes who would inevitably seek any advantage to win. The more undetectable the advantage gained, the better, and this brings us full circle to the issue of 'fair play' discussed in previous chapters. The IOC's justification for prohibiting certain doping substances does not rest upon the concept of 'fair play' or the extent to which the principle of fair play is violated by the competitive advantage provided by drugs. The IOC seems to have conceded that there is no such thing as 'fair play' in Olympic sport. Fair play is regarded as an ideal which cannot be realised in Olympic competition, and it is thus meaningless to try to incorporate it into the guidelines as a criterion for determining which performance-boosting substances are to be banned and which are not. As long as there are rich countries and poor countries, we are told, there can be no true measure of 'fair play', for the rich countries will by virtue of their wealth be able to provide training facilities, training opportunities, and technological advances of relevance to human performance not available to athletes from the poorer countries.

The IOC prohibition on drugs derives *not* from a consideration of unfair advantage, but from a consideration of the *harm* done by these substances, either to the athletes who take the substances or to other athletes who do not use the substances but who suffer say as a result of the aggressiveness of the athletes who do. Within the present context of deliberation the IOC's justification of guidelines seems at first blush convincing. However, technological innovations from genetic engineering are either now available or will soon be available that may provide athletes with a *harmless* and *undetectable* competitive advantage on the one hand, and the IOC with a new and more complicated challenge on the other. If the IOC prohibition on performance-boosting agents depends solely upon the concept of 'harm' as stipulated above, it is difficult to see, for instance, how a competitive advantage such as a bionic or genetically engineered eye used by an athlete in the shooting competition could legitimately be prohibited.

Although the field of bionics presents a number of interesting possibilities in regard to performance-boosting devices, I shall confine myself in the present chapter to an examination of certain developments taking place in genetic engineering which may soon make the drug problems now confronting the IOC, pale in comparison. I shall in what follows consider state of the technology aspects in regard to gene mapping, gene therapy using recombinant DNA techniques, and cloning, considering their potential relevance for improving sporting performance.

The birth of genetic engineering

Recent developments in biotechnology have given scientists the power to manipulate and control the biological destiny of every living thing on this planet. For the first time in human history, we have developed a technology which makes us masters of our own evolution. Medical science now has within its grasp the power to transform the evolutionary future of the planet, creating new life forms and irretrievably altering the genetic characteristics of others. Our technology has finally made us the architects of the gene pool itself, and the blueprints for the genetic future of humanity are in our hands. Such enormous power gives rise to many possible innovations and to a range of unprecedented applications, both within and without sport.

For the origin of the principles underpinning genetic engineering, we traditionally refer to an Austrian monk of the 19th century, Gregor Mendel, whose study of the inheritance patterns of the ordinary garden pea is regarded as having established the science of genetics. But it was a Swiss scientist, Johann Miescher, who, while investigating the nucleus of living cells, discovered an acidic compound with a peculiar molecular structure now known as DNA (deoxyribonucleic acid). However, the role which DNA played in passing on inherited characteristics remained a mystery until the 20th century.

In the 20th century, gene research intensified with the progressive shift of emphasis from cellular to molecular details. Toward the middle of this century, the theory of the gene as the basic building block of living organisms came to predominate, partly on the assumption that cellular processes could best be understood genetically. By the 1940s, the role which genes played by way of controlling the synthesis of enzymes and thus determination of hereditary traits was recognised, though the chemical structure of the enzymes, themselves protein constellations, was still enigmatic. In the early 1950s Linus Pauling elucidated the structure of the protein molecule, introducing the model of a coiled pattern in the shape of either a left-handed or right-handed helix as an appropriate description. The idea of a coiled helix had considerable explanatory power, and it was utilised by James Watson and Francis Crick to reveal the structure of DNA itself, the genetic material in the chromosomes. The results of their investigations came to public light in the publication of their celebrated article in the April 1953 issue of the scientific journal *Nature,* and their work was soon hailed as marking the inception of the genetic revolution.[1]

In that article Watson and Crick reported that the microscopic structure of DNA had the form of a helix not unlike Pauling's protein molecule, but in this case it was the model of a twisting double helix based on the idea of a spiral staircase. The steps of the spiral staircase structure were constituted by what were called 'base units'. Differences in genetic makeup depended, they claimed, upon the particular arrangement of base units which were composed of a modest sequence of four chemical nucleotides (i.e. adenine, guanine, cystosine and thymine). Often abbreviated by their first letters, A.G.C.T., these chemical substances have come to be referred to as the 'genetic alphabet'. Arranging the four letters in as many different configurations as possible, it was observed that there were 64 resulting genetic combinations, more than sufficient to produce the 20 fundamental amino acids, which in turn combine in a multitude of sequences to produce the entire range of protein variations manifested by living things. Generally speaking, the fewer the number of genes in combination, the simpler the form of the individual organisms, and vice versa.

Within a decade of their original discovery Watson and Crick had unravelled the mystery surrounding the basic mechanism through which DNA carries out self-replication and protein synthesis, and had uncovered the process by which genetic information is encoded in the chromosomes. The discovery was highly significant and paved the way for future developments in genetic engineering, as it showed how the genetic features of all living organisms, regardless of how complex, were encoded by the same chemical substances and governed by an identifiable code script. The genetic code having been broken, the engineering of hereditary characteristics within a particular genotype could now be undertaken systematically.

It was not until the 1970s, however, that the most radical and revolutionary development in genetic engineering occurred. To understand why it was revolutionary we need to remind ourselves that in a manner of speaking, the concept of genetic engineering, indeed, its practice, is not really new. Since the beginning of history, there have been persistent attempts to improve what nature had to offer us. We have long sought to improve the quality of grain, for example, and we have selectively bred animals, enhanced strains of flowers and hybridised fruits and vegetables. There have been some occasional and usually controversial attempts to engage in positive eugenics through the selective breeding of humans. Although we have in essence engineered particular genetic variations within species, however, we have virtually never engineered the genotypes of the species themselves. Until the 1970s, moreover, the boundaries between any two species were resolutely fixed and inviolable. While technology was adequate to permit the crossing of various strains of plants, it supplied no mechanism whereby it would be possible to cross humans and apes, or to introduce certain genetic characteristics of the one, say the strength advantage of apes, to the other. All this has now changed.

It is now possible to recombine DNA from altogether different organisms and to introduce new gene traits to replace the old. In the early 1970s Herbert Boyer of the University of California and Stanley Cohen of Stanford University succeeded in employing newly acquired knowledge of DNA to stitch together slices of genetic material from two completely unrelated species, thus actually creating new life organisms.[2] Referred to as 'recombinant DNA technology', this radically innovative form of genetic engineering has afforded the scientific capability required to combine features of wholly different organisms, to transfer genetic characteristics from one species to another, and even to edit the genetic code of an individual by reprogramming gene patterns which would previously have been unalterable and final.

Manipulating DNA in this way, or 'gene splicing' as it is now called, has momentous implications for the future of humankind in general and the future of sporting performance in particular. We have for the first time in the history of the human race the power to shape our own evolution, and we have the power to transform ineradicably our own genetic potential. Human and plant cells have already been successfully fused. Genetic engineering would seem to have the potential to make anabolic steriods utterly obsolete, for once the genetic disposition of a cell is altered, its subsequent processes are alleged to be as 'natural' as if it had not been altered. Let us approach these aspects more intently.

Gene mapping

A number of significant clinical triumphs have accompanied advances in genetic theory, encouraging the establishment of an applied commercial science of potentially staggering proportions. At the centre of any DNA molecule are sequences of paired bases which form various genetic messages. Sequences of base-pairs in triplicate are called 'codons' and provide the genetic program for the synthesis of a unique sequence of amino acids, joined by peptide bonds and thus known as 'polypeptide chains'. As a result of a series of remarkable biochemical processes, polypeptide chains are enfolded into the configurations which stand for specific proteins—such as protein constituents of enzymes, which figure in the regulation of metabolism.

By analysing the body's various amino acid sequences, it is now possible to mimic protein synthesis. Having broken the genetic code, it is possible to reprogram the genetic instruction encoded in the base sequences of DNA for the formation of protein itself. Each of the estimated 100 000 human genes (each accounting for approximately 1000 base pairs) contains within itself the total genetic program required for making a protein essential to a particular bodily function. It is thus possible in principle to repair dysfunctional genes by modifying the relevant nucleotides along the DNA molecule. Similarly, there is no logical reason why it should not be possible to alter the relevant nucleotide sequence in such a way that human genes are fashioned *de novo*. Identifying the chromosomal seat of particular genes is of course not one and the

same as the determination of exactly where on the chromosome
the gene is located, but enormous progress has been made in recent
years to ensure the accuracy of gene cartography.

Fragments of DNA can now be manipulated in a number of ways
to map gene sites. One technique known as '*in situ* hybridisation'
requires a copy or clone of the gene being traced. The copy is
labelled with a radioactive tag and then mixed with DNA from a
single chromosome or even part of a chromosome. Given the
double helix structure of DNA, any two strands of DNA closely
resembling each other will bind, as does the labelled gene with any
genetically relevant portion of the genome. This technique provides an accurate physical map of gene sites but is of limited use
in that it requires a copy of the gene in question.

Professor Leroy Hood, of the California Institute of Technology,
has developed an effective technique for sequencing larger pieces
of DNA.[3] Using a machine he calls the DNA sequenator, fluores-
cent dyes replace radioactive markers enabling geneticists to read
about 12 500 bases each day, and Hood claims that the current
reading figures could be improved tenfold. The technique known
as 'gel electrophoresis' permits larger pieces of DNA to be separated to determine trait locations expressed by 'restriction fragment
length polymorphisms' (RFLPs). Thousands of RFLPs have now
been mapped and identified. While this technique can separate
DNA fragments up to a few hundred bases long, the more sophisticated technique of pulsed-field gel electrophoresis (PFGE) facili-
tates the sequencing of fragments in the millions of bases long.[4]
One of the first genes mapped by the technique of linkage analysis
(a technique sponsored on the assumption that genes in physical
propinquity on a chromosome will tend to be inherited together)
was the gene responsible for a certain kind of colour blindness.

The potential application of genetic engineering techniques such
as these to bodybuilding is revolutionary, making the use of anabolic steriods and other bodybuilding drugs seem utterly archaic
and jaded. Consider for a moment the common problem of obesity.
It is estimated, for example, that nearly 35 million Americans are
overweight. Recent studies have demonstrated, however, that while
exercise and diet can serve to regulate weight, the disposition to
fatness is inherited.[5] What this means in physiological terms is
that the number and potential size of the some 30 to 40 billion fat
cells which figure in the human constitution are genetically programmed. Depending upon the nature of the genetic program, you
will have to exercise and diet more or less diligently to control your
weight. Indeed, for some individuals the state of being overweight

will, in genetic terms, be the normal state, and dramatic weight losses may thus be accompanied by systemic disruptions such as amenorrhea and pathological anorexia. Genetic engineering, coupled with in vitro fertilisation techniques, affords a revolutionary way to manage hereditary patterns of obesity. As we observed above, it is now possible to identify the chromosomal seats in virtue of which specific genetic traits derive. Utilising one of the gene-marking techniques described earlier, scientists recently managed to isolate the particular genes responsible for obesity predisposition in mice. Although mice have 40 chromosomes, as compared with 46 in humans, the experiments provided a sufficiently reliable proxy to extrapolate the genetic technique for human use, and scientists have now identified and cloned a gene for an enzyme responsible for fat storage. Commenting on this breakthrough, Professor Michael Schutz says, 'It is the key enzyme and key gene in the metabolism of triglycerides, which are the things laid down in the cells of fat people'.[6]

Indeed, experiments are now being undertaken which could well identify the *linkage-site* for the 'fat-forming' gene in humans, and it is not unlikely that a technique for reprogramming the gene responsible for the 'tendency to get fat' will be available within the next decade or so. Not only will hereditary obesity become a genetic indiosyncrasy of the past, but the example illustrates that it should be possible in the very near future to regulate the expression of virtually every major genetically induced characteristic, including complexion, eye and hair colour, male pattern baldness, height, bone structure, and body type in respect of muscle density.

To date, thousands of specific gene locations have been isolated, and a professor in Japan has made reasonable progress in building a calculating machine designed to optimise polypeptide sequences for molecules which exhibit specific genetic functions.[7] The discovery of an enormous array of restriction enzymes has made it possible to cut and splice any given strand of DNA at a point of particular gene expression within the appropriate polypeptide sequences. The recent discovery of a class of molecules called 'ligases', composed of other enzymes that speed up the process whereby cut DNA fragments are rejoined or spliced together with new genetic material has brought an even greater degree of control to the cell engineering process.[8]

Gene therapy

By inserting new instructions into the DNA base sequences via their host cells, scientists are able even to reprogram the number and potential growth pattern of muscle cells themselves. It is possible in principle, that is to say, to splice into the relevant cells of an adult human being a gene for muscle-cell augmentation which will then serve to reorganise the design program for the body's normal production of all subsequent cells of the same type. Revising genetic instructions which overrun hereditary characteristics in adult humans is extremely complicated, and the technique known as somatic 'cell modification' by which this reprogramming takes place has not yet been successfully accomplished with humans, though gene therapy of this kind has now been achieved in the context of remedying genetic deficiencies of some insects. The extension of such techniques to humans is thus less a matter of science fiction than one might suppose.

Recombinant DNA techniques have made possible another more radical approach to genetically engineered athletes, and there is evidence accumulating which suggests that these techniques can now be adapted for the purpose of programming muscular growth patterns in humans. It is important to distinguish this more radical approach of gene therapy techniques discussed thus far. The previous discussion of gene therapy spoke only of splicing together genetic material from the same species.

The more radical technique involves splicing genetic material from a particular species into a designated polypeptide sequence of a completely different species. The more radical technique entails what I shall call 'human hybridisation'. Even before the advent of recombinant DNA, techniques for the culturing of hybridised cells were first developed in the late 1960s. In 1967, researchers at New York University produced a hybrid culture of mouse and human cells.[9] It has only been in recent years, however, that recombinant techniques have become sufficiently sophisticated to sustain the level of gene manipulation required for gene therapy.

In 1981, Dr Thomas Wagner announced that the research team of which he was head had not only isolated the gene which partly regulated the manufacture of haemoglobin in rabbits, but had brought to term a mouse embryo into which the rabbit gene had been injected.[10] The resultant mouse was biologically unique, as the transferred rabbit gene which it contained produced its haemoglobin within the mouse as effectively as it had within the rabbit.

Another significant consequence of the hybridisation was that the heredity of the mouse had been altered permanently and passed on to subsequent generations. The biotechnological stage was thus set for the introduction of another genetically engineered mouse unlike any other mouse in history. This time, it was the rat growth hormone gene which was spliced into mouse embryos, some of which were then effectively brought to term. The resultant mice grew 2 to 3 times as fast as normal, and showed similar increases in both size and strength. In comparison, injections of rat growth hormone into adult mice have proved negligible in respect of size and strength gains. Capable of transferring their newly acquired characteristics to subsequent generations, these novel creatures have affectionately been dubbed 'supermice'. Since the engineering of supermice, considerable research has demonstrated that similar genetic manipulations, using the gene, for example, responsible for the manufacture of elephant growth hormone, afford the prospect of extraordinary size and weight increases in cattle and other animals reared for the commercial market.

It is clear that techniques of embryonic genetic engineering, generally known as 'germ cell modification', could in principle be employed to produce an athlete of considerable physical gifts. Indeed, scientists have actually developed a genetic engineering technique for the production of 'giant cells' capable of growing some 500 times larger than normal.[11] Using such techniques, it would be possible—though it is not now possible—to engineer the structure of muscle cells in ways which would far exceed the normal potential for muscle development. Germ cell modification of this kind, however, would have to be coupled with techniques of IVF or in vitro fertilisation. Such techniques are becoming increasingly more sophisticated and already make possible a range of germ cell modifications of potential relevance to human performance.

Cloning: something for the lonely athlete

If a superior individual—and presumably, then, genotype—is identified, why not copy it directly, rather than suffer all the risks, including those of sex determination, involved in the disruptions of recombination (sexual procreation). Leave sexual reproduction for experimental purposes; when a suitable type is ascertained take care to maintain it by clonal propagation
        (Joshua Lederberg, 'Experimental Genetics on Human Evolution', *Bulletin of the Atomic Scientists*, 1966.)

The dream of preserving and promulgating the best specimens within any species has a special relevance for human performance. While hard work is perhaps the ultimate key to athletic success, it is clear that genetic inheritance largely determines how hard one will have to work to achieve success. A bone structure such as Ben Johnson's or the length of stride exhibited by Flo Jo are extremely rare genetic gifts. The dream of cloning is the dream of being able to produce a carbon copy or copies of an already existent biological specimen. A clone of Arnold Schwarzenegger, for example, would entail the production of a new individual whose chromosomes are genetically identical to or duplicate of those of Arnold.

The dream of producing a superclone or of reproducing carbon copies of preferred biological individuals was until recently the prerogative of science fiction writers. In 1978, for instance, David Rorvik's book *In His Image* provoked controversy and outcry by suggesting that an American millionaire, code-named 'Max', sponsored the establishment of a research laboratory whose sole purpose was to perfect the technique of cloning a son for Max.[12] According to Rorvik, the research experiments were finally successful, and Max came to be the proud father of his own clone. Whether Rorvik's book was a hoax is not a subject I wish to dispute here. Whatever the outcome of that debate, it has now been superseded by the development of technology which has in fact transformed the science fiction of cloning into a reality. It is perhaps unsurprising that Rorvik prefaced his book, as I have prefaced this section, with a quotation from the Nobel Prize-winning geneticist, Joshua Lederberg, who in speaking of cloning, remarked: 'There is nothing to suggest any particular difficulty about accomplishing this in mammals or man, though it will rightly be admired as a technical tour de force when it is first accomplished. It places man on the brink of a major evolutionary perturbation.'[13]

Let us now consider more closely the somewhat bizarre possibility of producing athletic superclones. There are different ways in which cloning can be achieved. One type of cloning, it should be acknowledged, has long occurred naturally among some plants and animals. Natural cloning occurs when an unfertilised cell develops spontaneously into a living organism in which the chromosomes which constituted it are a product of the genetic code of a single genetic parent, thus bypassing the chance variation which results from sexual reproduction when the genetic codes of two individuals are combined. Natural cloning of this kind is referred to as 'parthenogenesis', deriving from the Greek word *parthenos*, which means 'virgin'. Examples of asexual reproduction can be found in a number of insects, including the wasp, the honeybee and the

greenfly. Dr Marlow W. Olsen of the Department of Agriculture
Research Center at Beltsville, Maryland affirms that turkeys can
occasionally reproduce through parthenogenesis, claiming to have
attended the hatching of several poults from unfertilised eggs.[14]

More extraordinary are reports that parthenogenesis even occurs
in human beings. Dr Helen Spurway, a geneticist from London
University College, alleges that one in every 1.6 million pregnan-
cies in humans results from parthenogenesis.[15] The explanation for
this remarkable phenomenon, several instances of which have been
reliably documented (see D.S. Halacy, Jr., *Genetic Revolution*[16], is
not entirely clear, but recent developments in holographic theory
have served to supply some important clues.[17] The basic idea is
that every body cell contains the genetic program for replicating
the entire DNA spectrum of the body. In the normal process of
development it is of course true that cells differentiate and special-
ise to assume various biological tasks; becoming, for instance, cells
of the eye, hair, skin etc. What holographic theory implies, however, is that the specialised function of a cell does not cancel or
destroy its potential for overall DNA replication. In other words,
specialisation of a cell is not incompatible with its potential for
assuming at different times and under different circumstances
other specialised functions. The DNA program for the specialised
functions of all cells is thus contained within every cell, masked by
the genetic emphasis upon one particular function rather than
upon some other. This being so, the explanation for human
parthenogenesis relies upon the possibility that a severe shock or
blow to the human body, or perhaps the experience of other forms
of intense emotional disturbance, is capable of triggering the acti-
vation of the full complement of the genetic program within a cell,
rather than a particular and singularly specialised aspect of it. A
dormant cell within the uterus, for example, could be jolted in
such a way that its potential for complete genetic replication is
activated, thus initiating the process of asexual reproduction or
what might be called a 'virgin birth'. The resultant child would in
every respect manifest a chromosomal pattern exactly as her
mother; the child would in fact be her clone. The product of such
parthenogenesis would, of course, necessarily be female.

Although parthenogenesis as described above produces clones,
natural cloning of this type is essentially a freak of nature. Cases of
deliberately induced parthenogenesis even outside the human
species are relatively rare. The few examples are noteworthy. At
the turn of the century the biologist Jacques Loeb discovered that
simply applying dry ice to an unfertilised sea urchin egg would
induce cloning.[18] In 1939 Dr Gregory Pincus was credited with

having induced parthenogenesis in a rabbit through the administration of thermal shock treatment,[19] and in 1952 Dr Robert
Briggs and Thomas J. King produced tadpole clones by genetically
manipulating a frog egg which had previously been fertilised.[20]
They first removed the nucleus of the egg—the central component
containing the genetic program of the female frog—and then
replaced it with tissue taken from another frog of the same species.
This research has been expanded by Dr J.B. Gurdon of Oxford,
who used ultraviolet radiation to destroy the nucleus of an
unfertilised egg cell of an African clawed frog.[21] Having enucleated
the unfertilised egg cell, he completed the cloning process by
implanting cells taken from the intestinal wall of the same frog.
With the addition of new chromosomal material the egg seems
somehow to have been tricked into functioning as if it had actually
been fertilised, thus growing into an exact replica of the original
African clawed frog.

Extending this cloning technique of nucleus transfer from
amphibians to humans is rather more complicated. The eggs of
amphibians, for instance, are relatively large, normally fertilised in
water and brought to maturity outside the body. In the case of
mammals (including humans) this is not the case. Nonetheless, in
1981 Karl Illmensee and Peter Hoppe were heralded as having
engineered the first successful nucleus transfer involving the cloning of a mammal.[22] Having removed the nuclei of a number of
mouse eggs, they replaced the genetic information of the original
nucleus with nuclei of cells taken from a 7-day-old mouse embryo.
Surrogate mouse-mothers into which the engineered eggs were
then implanted soon gave birth to genetically identical mice. To
date the technology required to clone human individuals from a
single cell which has been enucleated has not been developed,
though some reseachers such as Dr Kimball Atwood, professor of
microbiology at the University of Illinois, incline to the view that,
with a greater focus of resources directed toward this objective,
cloning could be a reality now.[23]

Nucleus transfer cloning, however, is not the only technique for
cloning. To appreciate the full impact of this other technique, we
need to gain some sense of the context in which it emerged and is
currently being employed. The kind of cloning which is already
possible has developed hand in hand with the invention of the in
vitro fertilisation technique or IVF, as it has come to be known.
The IVF technique is relatively straightforward but, as its full
desciption here would be extraneous to the present consideration, I
shall for now confine myself to describing only its initial stages.

Ovum or egg collection involves passing a hollow needle through
the vault of the vagina or percutaneously through the lower

anterior abdominal wall under ultrasonic visualisation and aspirating the ovum from a suitable ovarian follicle. The ovum is then deposited into a special solution which allows the egg to continue its maturation until it is ready to be fertilised. The semen is then added to the fluid containing the egg in the hope that a sperm will penetrate the egg.

On the assumption that the egg has been fertilised and gone through its first division, we are now in a position to bring about a novel kind of cloning. Under a microscope the newly fertilised egg appears as a two-cell embryo, and the first stage of cloning involves separating the two cells. Engineering the division of the embryo, it should be observed, simply duplicates the natural process of embryo cleavage which results in the development of identical twins. Inasmuch as their genetic constitution is identical, they are in essence clones of each other.

The success of the process of engineering twinned clones depends upon the fact that, for the first few days after conception, each cell is 'totipotent'. Each cell has, that is to say, the potential to divide and proliferate the complete range of cells that constitute a mature being of a specific genetic type. Given that the cells of an early embryo are undifferentiated (i.e. have not yet been genetically determined in the role of a specific type of cell) it is possible to extend the process of engineering twinned clones indefinitely. Once the separated cells themselves divide, the two-celled embryo can be divided yet again, adding another clone to the genetic stockpile.

It is to be admitted, of course, that this kind of cloning has limitations which nucleus transfer cloning does not. The cloning of twins, indeed even a large number of them, does not guarantee a carbon copy of an older person, so it would seem that we are still unable to replicate the superheroes of bodybuilding. This negative conclusion, however, would be mistaken. For it is currently possible to combine this form of cloning with embryo freezing, thus allowing a wide scope in respect of the actual age of clones produced by engineered division of the initial embryo. Embryo freezing is a very recent development, but it is an actual development. The world's first pregnancy utilising a frozen embryo was successfully carried out in Melbourne, Australia, in May of 1983 under the direction of the IVF team of Carl Wood.[24]

Embryo freezing makes possible a number of scenarios in which the current technique of cloning could be used to produce a genetic replica of an older person. Imagine, for example, that a number of clones are produced through engineered division of the original embryo and that the original embryo is implanted and brought to maturity, while the remaining clones are frozen. Several years might pass, providing sufficient time for the parents of the child to assess its intellectual, physical and personality traits. On the assumption that the parents were satisfied, they could then choose to have a cloned embryo thawed, implanted and brought to maturity as any normal sibling would be. The main difference, of course, is that these siblings are identical twins, but born years apart. The process could be repeated and, in doing so, a couple could rear a family of clones. Indeed, the situation becomes even more incredible when one considers that the embryos could remain frozen indefinitely. This means that the original child could grow to adulthood, become a Mr or Ms Olympia, and then decide to thaw one or more of the embryos in respect of which they are genetically identical. A Mr Olympia or Ms Olympia could thus choose to rear his or her clone as his or her own child. In the case of a Mr Olympia, the cloned embryo could be carried by his wife or a surrogate mother, if necessary. In the case of a Ms Olympia, she could be made pregnant with her own clone. The permutations are mind-boggling. Imagine that our original child grew to adulthood, got married and had children in the usual way, though a number of frozen clones could have been utilised for this purpose. Imagine now that upon reaching adulthood the children of our original child decide to rear their father's clones. This would in effect mean they would be rearing a genetically exact replica of their father, his clone, or their uncle, depending upon your feel for family relationships.

It has not been my aim in this piece to evaluate the moral propriety of cloning, but simply to show that cloning is not merely the idle conjecture of science fiction writers. Embryos are currently being frozen for a range of purposes, including those which I have sketched above. The making of an athletic superclone is not a futuristic dream; it is a current possibility.

The brave new world

Gene-splicers will make it possible for men to have babies and humans to eat hay. Once they accomplish this stuff, can bigger and better athletes be far behind? Let us consider the case of body-building.

To date bodybuilding has been concerned predominantly with maximising genetic potential in respect of what might be called 'quality muscular growth'. Ergogenic acids, including the use of anabolic steroids and other enhancement drugs, do little more than speed up and occasionally exaggerate the complex physiological processes by which food-protein is converted into muscle mass. While a bodybuilder may be able to increase significantly the size of his or her calves, the genetic program of the individual will ultimately determine whether it is long or short calves whose growth potential is being maximised. The same principle applies to shoulder width, length of biceps, width of hips and so on. When all the hard training and dieting are done, it is basically genetics which will legislate the law of successful outcome.

With the advent of genetic engineering has come the technological possibility of altering the genetic laws which govern successful bodybuilding outcome. Indeed, the range of possible genetic transformation is staggering. Once the Pandora's box of genetic manipulation is opened, however, it is not at all clear where the manipulation will stop. In their provocative book *Who Should Play God?* Ted Howard and Jeremy Rifkin allege that a major company in the US has been conducting genetic experiments to change the human digestive tract in such a way that humans, not unlike cows, could eat and digest hay.[25]

It is also claimed that certain of the genes of plants could be crossed with humans, thereby giving human skin the genetic character of a leaf capable of photosynthesis.[26] This would mean that the formation of carbohydrates from carbon and water in humans could be brought about simply from the action of sunlight on the chlorophyll in the genetically modified skin, thereby radically altering the need to eat. Research is also under way to modify even the human sense of smell.[27] The idea here is to render the sensory nerves in the nose that register unpleasant smells dysfunctional, while leaving the nerve centres for good smells intact. Given general environmental conditions and the existence of certain working conditions in which the smells of various pollutants have become overwhelming, it is argued that genetic manipulations of our sensory faculties may become commonplace.

Research undertaken by Dr Robert O. Becker of the Veterans' Administration Hospital in Syracuse, New York had shown that it is now possible to stimulate the partial regeneration of limbs in rats.[28] The hope is that this research could be extended to provide an engineering process for the regeneration of limbs and internal organs for humans. In the light of developments such as this, Nobel Prize winner Jean Rostand has been quoted as saying, 'it would be more than a game from the man-farming biologist to change the subject's sex, the colour of his eyes, the general proportion of body and limbs and perhaps the facial features.'[29] Other distinguished scholars believe that in the near future it will also be possible to implant a uterus in a human male's body, inducing gestation through artificial fertilisation or embryo transfer.[30] Inasmuch as men possess mammary glands, hormonal or genetic munipulations could be used to initiate the flow of milk from the male rudimentary breast. Women would no longer be biologically unique in having a monopoly on reproduction.

The possibility of genetically engineering a radically different body is no longer simply a science fiction fantasy. We have already observed that scientists can with varying degrees of sophistication synthesise cells, including 'giant cells' which possess the capacity to grow up to 500 times larger than normal. Moreover, present technology is sufficiently advanced to produce hybrid cells by fusing genetic material taken from two different organisms. Cell fusion has already been successfully undertaken, and experiments have shown that human cells can be spliced with the cells of a mouse as well as with the cells of a plant. We have also seen that current technology also provides for effective—though not exhaustive—'gene mapping' (i.e. determination of the location on the chromosomes of the specific genes responsible for physical traits such as skin pigmentation, hair and eye colour, height, etc.). Given that a number of specific gene sites can be identified, fusion techniques will soon enable the modification of the hereditary disposition of the gene by actually revising its original genetic program.

We have seen that nuclear transplantation and other techniques now make some forms of cloning possible. It may soon be technologically possible to clone our best athletes, and we could one day be confronted with a final heat of the 100 metres made-up largely of clones of previous gold medallists. Even more extraordinary is the technique of embryo fusion that involves the joining together of two individual embryos or fertilised eggs to ensure that the resultant human enjoys the genetic advantages of *four* biological parents rather than the traditional two. This means that it would be possible, using in vitro fertilisation techniques coupled with genetic engineering, to produce the human being who possessed the full genetic complement which would otherwise be derived from *four* separate individuals. The Brave New World of Bodybuilding offers a range of possible scenarios, and a number of actual scenarios such as genetically engineered endorphins.

The direction in which research on human genetic engineering is currently being pursued has, it should be observed, led primarily to attempts to eliminate 'bad genes'. Given that approximately 15 million Americans carry genetic disorders, wholly or partly determined as the result of defective chromosomes or genes, and that 80 per cent of all babies born mentally retarded are victims of diseases of genetic origin, it is no surprise that considerable effort is being made to advance this area of study.[31] The transition from the aim of eliminating genetic defects to the goal of making genetic

improvements such as the bodybuilder might seek amounts, I
believe, to the way one views two sides of the same coin, and this
in turn raises a number of ethical issues, some of which I should
now like to address.

The question of what a defect is and of what defects should be
eliminated is largely a matter of who is doing the defining and the
eliminating. This gives rise to questions of power and control and
the possible misuse of both. It is also interesting to observe that
the concept of a 'defect' acquires its negative force when viewed as
a condition we have no wish or need to tolerate. Inasmuch as
genetic engineering techniques afford the eradication of certain
defects, it follows that biotechnology ensures that there will be
fewer human defects we will have to tolerate. The paradox or
Catch-22 is, however, that traits we would have once quite will-
ingly tolerated, come in consequence of our newly acquired powers
to be regarded as defects. Our technological capability, in other
words, literally transforms the concept of 'defect' itself; technology
reshapes our values.

An IQ of 100, for example, would normally be considered
acceptable. Imagine, however, that recombinant DNA procedures
were used standardly to increase the IQ of all or most children to,
say, 150. This suggestion is not, by the way, as far-fetched as it
might at first seem. Experiments have shown that it is possible to
increase the brain size of a rat by as much as 76 per cent and to
bring about an equivalent increase in its learning capacity by
merely injecting the rat foetus with an appropriate growth
hormone.[32] Genetic engineering could also be used to bring about
the same result in the following way. The development of the brain
involves a process whereby the original cellular material undergoes
some 33 divisions to produce a brain of around 9 million cells.
Through genetic manipulation it is in principle possible to stimulate at least one further division, thereby doubling the number of
brain cells and their capacity for work.

Once the IQ of all or most children was genetically altered to
150, the otherwise acceptable IQ of 100 would come to be
regarded as unacceptable—it would be seen as a *defect*. What I am
trying to suggest here is that the technological capacity to eliminate 'bad genes' cannot be rigidly distinguished in practice from the
object of genetic improvement or 'positive eugenics', as it has come
to be called. The issue is not simply: 'If we are willing to eliminate
"bad" genes, why should we be unwilling to improve upon "good"
ones?' The issue is that genetic manipulation will by its very nature
alter irrevocably the concepts of 'good' and 'bad', the concepts of
'what is' and 'what is not' a defect. If we can genetically engineer
60 cm biceps, have we not devalued a 48 cm or even a 50 cm bicep

gained through 'honest labour'? One reply might be that this problem could be overcome by democratising the genetic base of competitive sport. To achieve this, we would ultimately engineer a hybrid athlete whose genetic character would reflect a range of preferred traits deriving from, say, the top-10 bodybuiders in the Mr Olympia or Ms Olympia lineup; then using the hybrid as a genetic template, clone a pool of potenial competitors, each of whom would have the same genetic chance of success as any other. If this were to happen, the standards of the competition would doubtless be extremely high but the contest would likely be somewhat boring. Part of what makes any competition exciting is that genetic variation provides for a kaleidoscope of diverse body types. Needless to say, judging a lineup of bodybuilding clones would be a nightmare. We would be looking simply to determine how well the competitors realised the *same* genetic potential.

A series of related issues is even more complex. If biotechnologists were to create such a hybrid, a genetic superperson, and then use it to clone other potential superpersons, to whom would such people belong? Who would be responsible for them? The first patent law in the US was passed in 1790 and was designed to protect the invention of virtually all items of manufacture. The question soon arose whether items of manufacture were by definition inanimate. A significant legal precedent was set in 1930 when Congress voted in favor of patent rights on plants produced through grafting, cutting and other modes of asexual production. The logical development of this legal disposition was extended at the turn of this decade when the Supreme Court approved patent rights on genetically engineered microorganisms, the basic presumption being that anything 'made by man' should admit of being patentable subject matter.

Within recent months the US Patent Office took the controversial step of extending patent rights to genetically engineered animals, including chimerical hybrids such as genetic crosses between different species.[33] The patenting of genetically altered human beings would seem to be the next logical step in this process. We could in fact find ourselves in a world in which commercial organisations set up research laboratories to breed a range of athletes, patenting for ownership purposes those deemed worthy to face the opposition. It may well be that genetic engineering will be used as the ultimate performance-boosting aid, and if no *harm* is done to an athlete in the process, what grounds does the IOC have in prohibiting performance-boosting transformations? Perhaps when all is said, the fundamental philosophy of sport must be capable of reinstating the concept of 'fair play' as a relative standard against which an unfair competitive advantage can be judged.

The ethical issues raised here—though hypothetical—are of staggering importance, and the way we resolve them will, I believe, make more of a difference than any of us might think to the kind of world—especially the sporting world—in which perhaps we and certainly our posterity will live.

9 Psychological parameters of drugs in sport
L. Scott Frazier

Mushrooms and herbs were used as drugs to increase performance in the ancient Greek Olympiads.[1] Aztec athletes made a potion from cactus that resembled strychnine, a stimulant used in the past by prize fighters.[2] Strychnine is a good example of a drug that has fallen into disfavour since even a slight overdose causes convulsions and death. However, the use of drugs in sports continues. In fact, in the past 20 years the problem has grown to epidemic proportions.

The study of drugs traditionally has focused on the physiological effects. The psychological consequences are less well known. This Chapter will bring together what today is understood to be the major psychological effects of drugs frequently used by athletes. Not that all of the drugs discussed appear on the IOC list of banned drugs. This is because a wider spectrum of drugs is used than those embraced by the IOC and its laboratories. Neither are all sports Olympic; in Australia the contact football sports have shown in 1991 evidence of 'social drug' usage as has been used in gridiron in the US for many years.

The structure of the Chapter is as follows: I will provide a working definition of a 'drug' in sport, distinguishing it from medication needed by athletes for legitimate medical conditions or diseases. I will discuss various classes of drugs in sports including: stimulants, depressants, sedatives, anti-anxiety agents and anabolic steroids. In each case, I will indicate their use, sketch their physical consequences; then focus on the psychological aspects. It will be shown that although there are some positive psychological consequences, the majority are negative and many are potentially severe.

Drugs in sport are associated with enhanced performance, and with the ideal of achieving a pinnacle of excellence. To many this is accompanied by concepts of prowess, vitality, not to mention fame and fortune. Drugs can enhance this quest but often the price is great. The scientific literature shows that in many instances there are long-term harmful consequences.

In some areas of drug abuse the statistics are encouraging. The use of cocaine, marijuana and amphetamines, at least in the US, seems to be on the decline overall.[3] Education, experience, parental and institutional concern, fear of detection, and interdiction all appear to be paying dividends. There is evidence, however, that drug use in sport in some categories is still on the rise. We will look at this evidence and ask 'why?'

Drug abuse

Athletes have colds and look for symptomatic relief; some suffer from conditions requiring regular medication. Diabetes is often given as an example. What sport official would want to limit insulin for an athlete—or a cup of coffee for that matter? Yet caffeine loading is banned. This raises a question: What is an acceptable drug and what is not? The European Council proposes the following as a definition of what is unacceptable: 'the administering or use of substances in any form alien to the body or of physiological substances in abnormal amounts and with abnormal methods by healthy persons with the exclusive aim of attaining an artificial and unfair increase of performance in competition'.[4]

With this definition it is possible to make an important distinction between the athlete who takes a cold remedy, an analgesic or anti-inflammatory for symptomatic relief or one who needs maintenance medication for an ongoing medical condition, from one who uses a substance or a procedure which has as its aim to confer an extra, unfair benefit. The distinction is between restoring or maintaining health versus bestowing an advantage.

This definition is helpful, but limited. It overlooks the issue of possible negative consequences of drug use. A drug is bad in direct proportion to its negative effects, physical and psychological. This principle applies not only to performance-enhancing drugs but also to substances used by athletes to help them deal with such things as anxiety, stress and tension. Depressants and anti-anxiety agents are abused by athletes as well as stimulants and anabolic steroids.

A more complete definition of drug abuse in sports should include not only the ethical issues such as unfair advantage but also whether the substance has negative side-effects.

Stimulants

Stimulants were probably the first drugs used in sports. An overdose by a Danish cyclist at the Rome Olympics of 1960 precipitated a campaign for their regulation. Today consistent routine checking at the level of world-class athletic competition has led to increasingly better control. For stimulants to be helpful they must be taken shortly before competition and they are easily detected.

It is understandable that where detection is less of an issue, for instance in high school and college athletic events, stimulant use is more widespread. By no means, therefore, has their use been eradicated in sport.

Caffeine

The most readily available stimulant is caffeine. Research indicates that at the lower levels of ingestion, caffeine acts as a mild stimulant. It is rapidly absorbed by oral administration. It activates the central nervous system and can decrease the perception of fatigue. There may be some nervousness and irritability noted with as few as two cups of coffee (250 mg).[5]

The US Olympic Committee considers excess caffeine a banned substance. To test positive an athlete would have to ingest the equivalent of six to eight cups of coffee (1.5 to 2 grams) three hours before testing. When the lower limits of intake, which vary from person to person, have been exceeded, negative psychological consequences occur.

Caffeine intoxication or 'caffeinism' is associated with the following symptoms: restlessness, nervousness, excitability, insomnia and gastrointestinal complaints. Further symptoms may include: muscle spasm, rambling flow of thought and speech, cardiac arrhythmia, psychomotor agitation and irritability. There may be mild sensory disturbances such as ringing in the ears. Higher doses (doses exceeding 10 grams), can cause grand-mal seizures, circulatory failure, and possibly death.[6]

After an athlete has relied on large doses of caffeine and wishes to withdraw, he or she may experience strong headaches accompanied by craving and depression. The depression may be long-lasting and can be complicated by tension, nervousness and irritability.

The potential benefits of caffeine are largely limited to endurance athletes. The physical plus psychological side-effects indicate that the disadvantages of caffeine-loading outweigh the benefits.

Amphetamines

Amphetamines and met-amphetamines ('speed') are more potent stimulants. They are difficult to detect in plasma but following oral administration, more than 50 per cent is excreted in the urine. Detectable amounts from as little as a single dose can be found in urine for as long as seven days.[7] Control therefore is quite easy if there are detection facilities.

The supposed beneficial effects of amphetamine use in sports is a strong subject of debate. Amphetamines have been popular with weight-lifters, wrestlers, jockeys and cyclists among others. These athletes take advantage of increased metabolism caused by the drugs in order to control weight in preparation for competition. Amphetamines are also used as 'endurance enhancers' during the competition itself although it is thought that all they do is mask various sensations of fatigue.

Amphetamines will produce, on a short-term basis, wakefulness, increased alertness, a heightened ability to concentrate on simple tasks, and an increased sense of initiative and confidence. Physiological effects include increased pulse and blood pressure, a higher metabolic rate, increased oxygen consumption and relaxation of the smooth muscles.

Since amphetamines were first synthesised in 1887, their use has been established in the treatment of various disorders including: obesity, narcolepsy, depression, hyperactivity in children, and fatigue. Athletes, as noted, want relief from fatigue, or at least want to mask the effects.

The problem with taking amphetamines is their marked negative side-effects. With use tolerance develops and although the mechanisms are unclear the anorexigenic and mood-elevating properties diminish. The development of tolerance necessitates an increase in the dose and consequently it is common for athletes to develop patterns of use which are compulsive.

A.J. Mandell[8] describes 'the Sunday Syndrome' associated with amphetamine abuse by professional American football players. Case studies document players who become arrogant, easily angered, irritable, inappropriately physically abusive (e.g. biting) and paranoid.

With increased frequency and use over time, the psychological effects of amphetamines become more pronounced. Initially an athlete might experience increased tension and nervousness but as use continues anxiety mounts. Feelings of unease turn to dread. Generalised fear may turn to paranoia.[9]

Prolonged use may lead to a particularly severe psychological state known as amphetamine psychosis.[10] The clinical pattern resembles paranoid schizophrenia. Individuals suffering from amphetamine psychosis may experience auditory and visual hallucinations, changes in sexuality with excesses and perversions, as well as thought confusion. As the syndrome progresses, symptoms become more severe with distortions in the sense of time, fear and an increase in aggression. There may also be delusions of persecution and ideas of reference. Further psychological and behavioural changes may include depression, anhedonia (apathy in the performance of acts which normally give pleasure) and social isolation.[11]

The symptoms associated with the withdrawal from amphetamines can also be serious. Individuals who are not strongly drug-dependent may be treated on an out-patient basis, but generally withdrawal should take place in a hospital or other treatment facility. The condition is generally marked by lethargy, headache, fatigue, nervousness, anxiety, nightmares and severe depression. Suicidal ideation is also a strong possiblity.

Cocaine

Cocaine, like the amphetamines, is a central nervous system stimulant. It is used by athletes as a mood-elevator, a confidence-enhancer, for increased alertness and to mask fatigue. At the turn of the century, cocaine was touted as a wonder substance. Freud prescribed it to his patients and he took it himself primarily to relieve depression.[12] Sir Arthur Conan Doyle, a physician, made his character Sherlock Holmes a user. Coca-Cola had it as a central, original ingredient. Earlier US presidents have been known to rely on it: William McKinley for example. Cocaine has legitimate medical uses. It continues to be an effective local anaesthetic.[13]

Cocaine, of course, has been and still remains a major drug of abuse. However, its use in certain populations is presently declining. A recent survey shows that in the United States from 1987 to 1988, the overall proportion of high school seniors who used cocaine at least once decreased by one-fifth. Use of cocaine within the last 30 days — defined as 'current' use — among high school seniors declined from 4.3 per cent in 1987 to 3.4 per cent in 1988. A similar decrease in cocaine use was found in US college populations. Here use fell from an overall 17 per cent to 10 per cent. This trend was noted among young adults also aged 19 to 29 years.[14]

Although there is no specific information concerning current levels of cocaine abuse among athletes, it may be safe to suppose that a reduction in use could well be occurring among this population as well. The physical and psychological effects of cocaine are well documented, and it is a good idea to see them as interrelated. During cocaine intoxication, the cerebral cortex is stimulated. Psychologically this is often accompanied by feelings of increased strength, euphoria, optimism, and quickness of thought. There are marked negative psychological side-effects, however. These include feelings of restlessness, tension, irritability, excessive excitation and problems with memory.

Users find that the initial euphoria is quickly replaced by a depressive effect. The reason for this is that the stimulation brought about by cocaine is quickly followed by decreased central nervous system functioning. This process sets into motion a destructive cycle. To alleviate the depressant effect, the user often turns immediately back to cocaine in order to recapture the earlier 'high'. The result is re-use of cocaine to mask the negative effects of cocaine itself.

Reverse tolerance is a further complicating issue. With increased use there is increased sensitivity. Negative symptoms become more pronounced with the same dose. Agitation turns to marked anxiety. Loose mental associations lead to thought confusion. Paranoid ideation may increase, with auditory and visual hallucinations.

The American *Diagnostic and Statistical Manual of Mental Disorders* (3rd rev. ed.) summarises the symptoms of cocaine intoxication: 'euphoria, fighting, grandiosity, hypervigilance, psychomotor agitation, impaired judgement, and impaired social or occupational functioning'. Other specific signs may include 'tachycardia, pupillary dilation, elevated blood pressure, perspiration or chills, nausea, vomiting and visual or tactile hallucinations.'[15]

Withdrawal from cocaine causes numerous psychological symptoms. These include depression, paranoia, tension, irritability, nervousness, upset and suicidal ideation. In withdrawal, the craving for the drug increases.

Treatment of cocaine dependency is complicated and usually expensive. The most successful programs involve a multi-modality approach within a structured environment. Successful treatment usually incorporates support, guidance, education and structure with social, family, peer and medical-psychiatric input. The treatment of acute cocaine intoxication may include the use of short-acting barbiturates, later incorporating anti-depressant or anti-psychotic medication to counteract the symptoms of withdrawal.

Depressants

Depressants are used by athletes either to counteract a stimulant taken earlier or as a strategy to deal with stress, particularly the pressure of self-expectations, the wishes and desires of coaches, parents, peers and the public.

Alcohol

Athletes shy away from alcohol before an event. They are aware of the adverse effects on performance including decreases in reaction time, hand-eye coordination, accuracy, balance and gross motor skills.[16] Following a sport event, when it is time to relax or 'party', or in preparation for sleep, many athletes engage in alcohol abuse. Some feel that alcohol is a 'safe' drug. Perhaps for this reason, it is the most abused of the central nervous system depressants.

With marked alcohol intoxication changes occur. A person's usual behaviour is accentuated or altered. In some instances the alterations may be encouraged. For example, a shy person might become loquacious and more social. However, intoxication brings with it maladaptive behaviors. Impaired judgement and decreased reaction time sometimes cause traffic fatalities, boating mishaps, drownings and sportmobile accidents. In the US, one-half of all highway fatalities involve alcohol. More than one-half of all murders are believed to be associated with intoxication.[17]

The initial euphoria associated with drinking soon changes as the early 'disinhibitory' phenomena give way to irritability, emotional lability, impaired social, occupational and athletic functioning. A major emotional by-product of alcohol abuse is depression. Often the abuser 'self-medicates' for the symptoms of alcohol abuse with alcohol, seeking the earlier euphoric state. But this is short-lived and the process sets up a self-defeating cycle of ingestion, heightened state, negative effects, depression, followed by re-ingestion. Approximately one-fourth of all suicides in the US occur while a person is intoxicated.[18]

By the time this destructive cycle is apparent, an athlete will find that his or her sporting performance has been negatively affected. By then the road to recovery is arduous. Athletes who have been drinking to self-medicate for anxiety or depression may benefit from minor tranquillisers or anti-depressants. But these cause other concerns especially since concurrent alcohol use might modify their effects. Other treatment modalities for alcoholism include aversion therapy, systematic desensitisation, hypnosis, psychotherapy and social support systems such as Alcoholics Anonymous.

Sedatives and anti-anxiety agents

Athletes are often prescribed sedatives and anti-anxiety agents to help them deal with stress. The medical sanction for the drugs makes their use preferable to alcohol. Negative effects, however, do exist and there is a strong potential for dependence and tolerance. Sedative-hypnotics help to ease tension and promote rest. A good night's sleep is a valuable commodity prior to a sporting performance. For many athletes it is elusive and so the temptation to rely on drugs to aid sleep may be strong.

Sedative-hypnotics depress the central nervous system and affect the cerebral cortex, limbic system, hypothalamus and ascending reticular formation. They appear to inhibit neurotransmitter release and to interfere with neurotransmission at the post-synaptic membrane. They have an additive effect when used with alcohol or other drugs, making them especially dangerous. Tolerance develops as well as physical dependence. With abrupt withdrawal, general depressant withdrawal syndrome can arise. Abstinence following addiction can be potentially life-threatening and may require intensive hospitalisation. Early symptoms associated with abstinence include agitation, anger, anxiety, nausea and vomiting. Later, there may be tachycardia, abdominal cramps and hypotension. Seizures may then develop. Delirium occurs 50 per cent of the time with seizures. Exhaustion and cardio-vascular collapse may end the athlete's life.

Examples of sedatives commonly abused include:

• Nembutal (pentobarbitone) and Seconal (secobarbital). These drugs are used primarily for their sedative-hypnotic properties. They are strongly subject to abuse. Tolerance builds rapidly both in the liver and the CNS. Strong physical dependence develops and depression is a common side-effect in the course of use and after abstinence. Suicide due to and with these drugs has been noted.

• Choral hydrate: This is the oldest and best known sedative-hypnotic. It induces sleep at low doses without affecting REM sleep patterns. Tolerance builds quickly with habitual use. Physical dependence is also a significant problem. Depression with decreased levels of overall energy is associated with use and delirium has been noted with abrupt withdrawal.

• Quaaludes (methaqualone). Quaaludes have been used by athletes primarily as a 'recreational' drug. The reason for this is that the drug acts directly on the central nervous system but does not affect the reticular activating system, the medulla or the midbrain. For these reasons, it has a calming, yet intoxicating effect without immediately inducing fatigue or a desire for sleep. Although the initial primary effect is hypnotic, there have been instances where subjects reported restlessness and anxiety.[19]

It has been estimated that approximately 2 grams a day taken over a period of four weeks may produce physical dependence. Prolonged use yields depression associated with lethargy and diminished initiative. It is common for there to be hangovers after its use. Abuse is usually complicated since methaqualone is often taken along with other substances especially alcohol. An overdose can be fatal. (The usual dose is 150 to 300 mg; a lethal dose varies between 8 and 22 grams).[20]

In addition to sedative-hypnotics, anti-anxiety agents are used by athletes to deal with tension and pressure associated with the exigencies of sport. These agents can be divided into two subclasses: first, benzodiazepines such as Valium (diazepam) and Librium (chlordiazepoxide); second, barbiturates and carbamates such as Miltown (meprobamate). Beta-blockers are also used in the treatment of anxiety.

Of these substances, the barbiturates are the more toxic and addictive and produce more severe CNS depression. The barbiturates have no particular advantage as far as an anti-anxiety agent is concerned and therefore the benzodiazepines and meprobamate are preferred.

In general, these compounds have less abusive properties than the sedative-hypnotics and barbiturates. Five times the therapeutic dose over a considerable period of time, probably 3 to 4 months, is required for physical dependence. There is, however, a strong tendency toward psychological dependence. Overdose leading to death is significantly less common.

As a class, these anti-anxiety agents have been very much overprescribed. 'Open-ended' prescriptions to athletes have been common. Their primary negative psychological side-effect is depression. With use over time, depressive symptoms increase eventually inhibiting training and decreasing performance during the sporting event. Often the athlete is not aware that his or her decreased drive is due to the drugs. He or she may see it as a 'slump'. Precisely because the symptoms of abuse in this instance are not acute, they may often go undiagnosed. The athlete may then try all manner of motivational aids to 'get out of the slump', when what is needed is to drop the medication.

With each of the sedatives and anti-anxiety agents there is a pattern that often develops. The athlete usually obtains the drug by way of prescription for treatment of insomnia or anxiety. He or she then gradually increases the dose, justifying this as legitimate treatment for symptoms. As the desire and need for the drug become greater, the athlete turns to a number of different doctors in order to obtain sufficient supplies.

Negative side-effects ensue. The individual finds that he or she becomes preoccupied with obtaining the substance. There is eventual interference with performance in social, academic, occupational and athletic areas. At this point, the athlete becomes alarmed and hopefully seeks help.

Beta-blockers

Athletes have used beta-blockers to help them remain calm and to treat performance anxiety. The process by which these substances work is complicated and not fully understood. There are what is know as beta 1 receptors in the heart, kidneys and adipose tissue. Beta 2 receptors are found in the liver, bronchi and arteries. Beta-blocking medication actually closes off some of the receptor sites keeping out stimulating agents that the body produces. In this way, body processes and behaviour are altered.

There are many medical uses for beta-blockers including the treatment of cardiac arrhythmia, hypertension, migraine headaches and the management of various mental problems including schizophrenia and anxiety states.

Athletes may be prescribed beta-blockers to deal with a medical problem, often anxiety. Beta-blockers have also been used to help athletes who have special needs for control. Beta-blockers can calm the heart rate thus increasing accuracy in events such as rifle and pistol shooting or archery. (Musicians may use beta-blockers to control performance anxiety.) A beta-blocker, however, adversely affects endurance, therefore, it is not indicated in an event where energy production is required as well as control such as the biathlon which incorporates cross-country skiing and marksmanship.

The negative psychological effects vary from beta-blocker to beta-blocker. A study of these adverse effects, however, yields some symptoms which are relatively universal. They include: lightheadedness, depression, vivid dreams, hallucinations, disorientation, emotional lability, memory loss and fatigue.[21] Of course not all athletes using beta-blockers will experience these symptoms;

however, the potential for their emergence is significant and must be factored into any decision whether their use is warranted. Also, use must be closely monitored.

Anabolic steroids

Cocaine and marijuana abuse at least in the US seems to be on the decline; the use of anabolic steroids, however, is reaching epidemic proportions.[22] Athletes and non-athletes are experimenting in record numbers.

For over 30 years, athletes have used anabolic drugs. Anabolic steroids are derivatives of testosterone which are either injected directly into the body or consumed orally in tablet form. Because steroids are rapidly metabolised by the liver, and in quantities do damage to it, the preferred method of delivery is through injection.[23] In cases of abuse, it is not uncommon that steroids will be taken along both avenues, orally and by injection.

Many athletes will engage in questionable behaviour if they believe that by doing so they can establish a competitive advantage. Many believe the use of anabolic steroids provides a 'winning edge'. It is felt by some that presently it is necessary to take steroids in order just to compete, and that their not doing so would place them at a distinct disadvantage.

Controversies surround anabolic steroid use. A central question is whether steroids in fact improve athletic performance. The number of athletes using them would indicate a strong belief that their performance is improved. What is clear is that despite the debate, the number of athletes taking anabolic steroids is significant and growing.

In 1985, it was estimated that one million US athletes were taking anabolic steroids.[24] Today that number would have to be multiplied many times over. A feeling for the depth of this issue comes from recent research conducted by Buckley, et al.[25]

Dr Buckley and his associates reviewed the literature on anabolic steroid use. In 1973, a study of five American universities found that 1.5 per cent of the college population, including women, were anabolic steroid users. Just two years later, in 1975, another study showed that 4 per cent of the athletes at Arizona high schools used steroids. In 1986, a study based in Minneapolis found that at one high school 8 per cent of high school senior males indicated they had used steroids.

Buckley's recent study establishes the estimated prevalence of anabolic steroid use among high school seniors nationwide in the US. Subjects were 12th-grade male students in both public and private high schools. The sample of schools was drawn from a pool of 150 high schools in various parts of the nation. A major criterion for a school's participation was that it had a certified athletic trainer. This narrowed the sample population to 10 per cent of all high schools in the country.

The results were striking: 6.6 per cent of 12th grade male students were using or had used anabolic steroids. Of this group, 47.1 per cent of the users participated in school-sponsored sports, specifically football and wrestling; however, 26.7 per cent of the group which used anabolic steroids did not participate or intend to participate in sports at all.

In Buckley's study of those who used anabolic steroids, 57.8 per cent felt that their strength was 'greater than average'. Also, 39.7 per cent of those who used anabolic steroids reported their overall health as 'excellent'. This corresponded with only 24.1 per cent of non-users. This statistic is made all the more significant when the consequences of anabolic steroid use are taken into consideration. It would seem to indicate that users feel that anabolic steroids help promote health when in fact scientific studies show the opposite.

The research also set out a profile of adolescent use. It found that more than one third of users (38.3 per cent) stated that they first used anabolic steroids at the age of 15 or younger. A second third started their use before the age of 16. These findings would indicate that it is not uncommon for users to begin as early as seventh grade. Information from southern California indicates that use presently is widespread in this age group.

According to Buckley et al. only 18.2 per cent of the users reported having taken but one cycle. Almost 40 per cent of them indicated that they had done five or more cycles of use. 'Stacking' of drugs—using more than one anabolic steroid at the same time—was relatively widespread. The study found that approximately 44 per cent took more than one type of anabolic steroid at the same time; 38.1 per cent stated that they had used anabolic steroids both orally and by injection.

When asked the reason for taking these drugs, most (47.1 per cent) indicated that it was 'to improve athletic performance'. However, a strong second reason was the improvement of 'appearance'. As noted earlier, 26.7 per cent of the group indicated that this was a main reason for use.

Concerning their sources, the user group indicated that the black market accounted for 60.5 per cent. Approximately 20 per cent of the users, however, indicated that their primary source was a health care professional (defined as a physician, pharmacist or veterinarian).

This is the first nationwide study of anabolic steroid use in the US among male adolescents. There are no statistics available concerning equivalent nationwide female use. The study concludes that the population at risk is broader than previously thought. The study dealt two major surprises. First, it was not realised that anabolic steroid use began at such an early age. Second, although it was recognised that use was growing, most had the impression it was for supposed increased benefits in athletic competition. The study points out that 'appearance' is a strong reason for many to take steroids. In southern California, this reason may actually supersede the supposed athletic gains that are obtained. Buckley et al. note that their findings are probably conservative and under-represent the real situation.

There is less accurate information with respect to anabolic steroid use among athletes beyond high school. Today, we must rely on surveys which are not always rigorous and the testimony of users and former users for information concerning this group.

It is estimated that more than 80 per cent of national and international male bodybuilders, weight-lifters and participants in the shotput, discus, hammer and javelin-throws have used anabolic steroids.[26] American football players, especially linemen, use anabolic steroids frequently. The sprinter, Ben Johnson, admitted that he took anabolic steroids and other banned performance-enhancing substances beginning in the early 1980s up until the time he tested positive in the 1988 Summer Olympics at Seoul.

Two East Germans prominent in international sports recently claimed that athletes in their country were required to take banned chemicals. Hans-George Aschenbach, a four-time world champion ski jumper and a gold-medal winner in the 1976 Winter Olympics, charged that performance-enhancing drugs including anabolic steroids were administered to athletes as early as age 13. Steroids, he contends, were used in sports such as skiing, swimming, figure skating, gymnastics and of course, in the power sports. This study was corroborated by Hans-Jurgen Noczenski, former chairman of the East German Judo Federation.

It is apparent that women athletes are becoming more ensnared in the web of drugs. For some time females were assumed not to use drugs extensively with only few exceptions. Presently this appears not to be the case. The US National Collegiate Athletics Association found that there is little difference in the pattern of drug use and abuse between male and female athletes.[27] Although there has not been a comprehensive national survey of female athletes, anecdotal accounts suggest that the prevalence of drug use

among women athletes is high. Sports most associated with anabolic steroid use in females are bodybuilding, power-lifting, track
and field as well as swimming.

The effects of anabolic steroids
The personal accounts of athletes indicate that the physical and
psychological effects of steroids are significant. Anecdotal information is substantiated by statistical research.

Diane Williams is one of the first Olympic athletes to confess
publicly to steroid use. In an interview with America's ABC-TV
(July 1989), she stated that she did experience muscle growth but
it was associated with increased hair. She found that the appearance of a mustache and a beard troubled her greatly. In addition,
she experienced internal gynaecological problems along with pso-
riasis. Also, she stated there were profound psychological effects.
She felt that she was 'worth nothing'. There was an overall feeling
that she was 'less than a human being'. Her sense of de-
humanisation was tied to feelings of depression and despair.

More dramatic effects have recently been noted by Tommy
Chaikin, a lineman at the University of South Carolina.[28] Following extended anabolic steroid use, Chaikin found that he suffered
from strong anxiety attacks. He felt he was losing control. Nightmares affected his sleep and depression stalked him. He began to
feel more and more discouraged and suicidal. Eventually it was
necessary to hospitalise him and to treat him with anti-psychotic
and anti-depressant medication.

Initially, the effects of the steroids were positive. He noted that
he was more motivated in the weight room and because of the
increased energy and positive reinforcement from accelerated
muscle growth he worked harder. His sex drive increased phenom-
enally; however, with time he began to feel strange and on 'edge'.
He developed aggression that eventually frightened him. His
temper was short. He found himself getting into fights and his
ferocity was alarming. 'I was beginning to feel like a killer', he
stated. 'I don't know if I could call steroids addictive', he said, 'but
there is a vicious cycle involved with using them. The growth of
the muscles enhances the aggression and other physical changes
caused by the drug, and those changes, in turn, make you want to
get bigger and take more steroids. Plus, there is a terrible let down
when you come off them. I would be very high and there would be
this extreme depression. And after each cycle, the come down itself
would get worse.'

Chaikin noticed strong personality changes. He found that his
behaviour was erratic. He stated that images of violence often filled

his mind. 'I drive along and find myself thinking about sick things like crushing people to death, tearing off their limbs. I'd be grinding my teeth and gripping the wheel so hard that my arms would hurt.'

Anxiety attacks led to feelings of being out of control. Paranoia set in. Thoughts of suicide were powerful. Eventually he put a gun to his head in his university room. Fortunately he was able eventually to manage his symptoms with the help of hospitalisation, anti-psychotic and anti-depressant medications followed by psychotherapy.

Controlled, statistical studies presently are beginning to corroborate such anecdotal accounts.

Animal experiments indicate that high testosterone levels promote irritability and aggression against unfamiliar males. High testosterone is also associated with aggressive behaviour in teenage boys. Research in Sweden indicates that it is the high testosterone level that leads to aggression rather that vice-versa.[29]

The most comprehensive account of psychological effects associated with anabolic steroid use comes from Pope and Katz.[30] In order to explore the consequences of anabolic steroid use, they recruited and interviewed 41 bodybuilders and football players who used the drugs. The subjects ranged from 17 to 51 years and included 39 men and two women.

Their observations suggest that the medical literature may have underestimated the effects of anabolic steroids in that the muscle gains by the subjects were dramatic. There were, however, associated physical problems noted by the users including: acne, temporary testicular atrophy, excessive development of mammary glands in males (gynaecomastia), difficulty urinating, hair loss, and in both of the women, deepening of the voice.

The psychological consequences were striking: 12.2 per cent of the subjects displayed psychotic symptoms; 22 per cent of the subjects developed a full affective mood disorder. Over one out of every three of the users had strong diagnosable psychiatric symptoms. None of the subjects had symptoms during periods of no steroid exposure.

Of the subjects with psychotic symptoms, there were noted auditory hallucinations, paranoid delusion, delusions of reference, and grandiose delusion. Additional subjects reported further psychotic symptoms such as paranoid jealousy, mild referential thinking and pronounced grandiose beliefs. Each of the users who experienced the psychotic symptoms was taking between two and four different kinds of steroids.

The 12.2 per cent of the subjects who met the DSM III-R criteria for a manic episode had characteristic symptoms which included a distinct period of abnormally elevated expansive or irritable mood. During the mood disturbance, various abnormalities were noted including inflated self-esteem, decreased need for sleep, loquaciousness, flight of ideas or thoughts, distractibility, increase in goal-directed activity, psychomotor agitation and excessive involvement in activities which have a high potential for painful consequences (e.g. sexual indiscretions). No-one reported a manic episode when there was no exposure to steroids.

In addition, 12.2 per cent developed a major depression during withdrawal from steroids. Only one user had a previous history of major depression. Therefore, overall 22 per cent developed full affective syndrome during episodes of steroid use or while withdrawing from it.

Pope and Katz state that their findings should be considered descriptive rather than quantitative. They are under the impression that only a minority of steroid users were willing to be interviewed and thus the percentages are probably conservative.

The authors noted that psychological effects of anabolic steroids are not easily studied. They found that the doses used by their subjects were often ten to 100 times higher than those used in medical studies. Also, their subjects 'stacked' as many as five or six different drugs. Finally, the athletes were disinclined to indicate the specifics of steroid abuse to the researchers. It may also be that athletes are not fully aware of the kinds of drugs they were using and their dosage.

It is probable that the negative psychological effects of steroids for female athletes is greater than for males. The reason for this is that the changes that occur with anabolic steroids for females are ego-dystonic. That is, the changes are at odds with a female's basic gender characteristics.

When anabolic steroids are used by women there are virilising effects. Hair growth appears on the cheeks, upper lip and chin. Baldness may occur, breasts shrink, and perhaps what is most disturbing, the voice deepens. The facial hair, baldness and deepening of the voice are often irreversible.[31]

Female athletes find it hard enough to establish their identities in a world that is based on competition and is traditionally male dominated. The 'masculinisation' of a female's body causes additional psychological conflict.

Why, with such marked physical and mental consequences is steroid use increasing? Why is it not falling off like the use of cocaine, marijuana, amphetamines, quaaludes, and other drugs?

One reason is the perception by athletes that steroids work. Ben Johnson did win the 100 metres race in a world record time of 9.79 seconds. It can be argued that anabolic steroids did not hurt his performance. Presently, the scientific literature may not accurately reflect the edge that steroids give, at least in certain sports. Anabolic steroids have their source in medical treatment. Athletes perceive that they do confer powers with training that are attained more quickly and that surpass non-users. A person 'looks' bigger, stronger and healthier after having taken them. Increased performance and appearance give a persuasive 'rationale' for continued use.

Most athletes are adolescents or young adults. Denial and tendency to 'live for the moment' are characteristic of these populations. The research by Buckley et al. shows that users wrongly but strongly hold a perception that steroid use provides benefits which promote health. When presented with evidence which counters their beliefs, users often criticise the data-base and motives of the expert.

Athletes do not necessarily consider the increased aggression associated with steroid use as negative.[32] On the contrary, it is viewed as a force pushing toward excellence. Other mood changes associated with steroid use are either denied or their consequence minimised. Interestingly, it is often the girl- or boy-friends of athletes who first become alarmed and seek information. The users have a tendency, if they recognise the symptoms, to ascribe them to other stressors e.g. work, school, finances etc.

Most athletes derive their information on steroids from popular trade magazines, peers and 'gym gurus'.[33] Few have medical input. When scientific information is presented, if conflicting, there is a strong tendency to discount it. Denial plays a strong role.

For these reasons, treatment is complicated. In general, classical drug treatment programs for other abuses such as cocaine are inadequate.

Conclusion

Drug abuse by athletes is widespread. The harmful consequences of various drugs have not been fully appreciated by athletes.

Stimulants lead to tension, anxiety, nervousness, irritability with depression. Dependency is a problem and tolerance is easily established. Psychosis resembling paranoid schizophrenia can result from excessive amphetamine use.

Depressants including alcohol, the sedative-hypnotics and anti-anxiety agents are used by athletes to 'medicate' in order, they think, to deal better with stress. Again dependency and tolerance are significant problems. During use and especially in withdrawal the result is often a depressive state—clinical in nature—which can lead to suicidal ideation, intent and sometimes action.

Anabolic steroids are perhaps the most pernicious of all the drugs. They are associated with strength, athletic prowess and health. However, their negative psychological effects are marked. Athletes on steroids have become tense, nervous, irritable, highly aggressive, combative, seemingly impervious to pain, self-destructive and suicidal. Mania, depression, and psychotic features have emerged with use.

Athletes are not receptive to these findings. They have an exceedingly strong will not just to survive but to excel. A 'magic pill' is hard to throw away.

Athletes, by and large, are adolescents or young adults, interested in immediate results, often minimising future consequences. Bodies are seen as machines to be manipulated—something to be experimented with. They find it hard to think about the possibilities of life in their thirties or forties with damaged livers, premature baldness and susceptibility to or actual experience of psychiatric disorders. Also, athletes have strong authority figures tacitly or specifically emphasising success, sometimes at any cost. Parents, coaches, doctors, peers, spectators, all encourage that extra effort. Unfortunately, the athlete often turns to the bottle for the 'extra edge'.

These issues make intervention extremely difficult. Traditional drug treatment centres are usually not effective. What is needed is a multi-modal approach incorporating, among other things, the very people to whom the athlete initially has turned for guidance: parents, coaches, doctors, and peers. All must be informed of the dangers of drugs: physical and psychological.

10 Medical effects and side-effects of ergogenics in athletes
Bob Goldman

> The merciless rigor of modern competitive sports, especially at the international level, the glory of victory, and the growing social and economic rewards of sporting success (in no way any longer related to reality) increasingly forces athletes to improve their performance by any means possible. (Manual on Doping, Medical Commission— International Olympic Committee.)

As the emerging speciality of sports medicine grows it is critical that physicians become more aware of the extensive use of drugs by athletes. The desire by athletes to enhance their performance is a strong one, and in the climate of the financial, as well as social, benefits of sporting success, the desire to succeed overrules ethics, as well as healthy logic. The use of synthetic or other banned substances and techniques in sports is not a new one and it will take a comprehensive program to control and alleviate sports drug use.

It is the moral duty of all those involved with athletes, and who care for the healthy future of competitive sport, to ensure that it is 'drug-free'. All young children participating in the sport must grow with the certain knowledge that they can improve their performance naturally, and that if they choose to compete, it will be on the basis of fair comparison.

The purpose of this Chapter is to engender an understanding amongst physicians as to the physical danger and moral wrong of doping. By a process of education, doping can be diminished and finally eradicated. Physicians through their leadership are capable of influencing, for example, athletes, teachers, coaches, other sports physicians and youth leaders.

The deliberate use of drugs to enhance sporting achievement is known as 'doping' and is considered cheating. Of course, drug use in the athletic community is not merely a contemporary phenomenon, but originated with sport itself.

Greek wrestlers of ancient times were thought to eat five kilograms of lamb per day to increase strength, and the distance runners of that time believed sesame seeds increased their endurance. Others drank a mixture of strychnine and wine, while others ate hallucinogenic mushrooms to mentally prepare for competition. The Berserkers, ancient Norse warriors, fought in a frenzied state under the influence of psychoactive mushrooms.

The earliest reports of drug-taking by athletes in competition in modern times were in Amsterdam in 1865, when swimmers in canal races were charged with taking dope. It was also about that time that the first evidence of doping among cyclists appeared. In 1869, the coaches of teams of bicycle racers were widely known to be administering the heroin-and-cocaine mixture now known as 'speedball' to increase the endurance of their racers. The practice caught the attention of the sports world when the first recorded drug-related death in sports befell a cyclist in a race in 1886.

Drug-taking in sports cropped up repeatedly through the end of the 19th century and on into the 20th. The Belgians were said to be taking sugar tablets soaked in ether, the French to be taking caffeine tablets, and the British to be breathing oxygen and taking cocaine, heroine, strychnine and brandy, all in attempts to gain the competitive edge.

The fascination with the male hormone has intrigued man for centuries, as the testes were viewed as the seat of man's power and virility. In 1894 Berthold performed experiments on the growth of combs and wattles in fowl (roosters) which predated the science of endocrinology by half a century. He removed the testicles from four roosters, making them capons, and then opened the bellies of two of the sexless birds and reimplanted one testicle. The implants took hold, and while the two castrated roosters became fat pacifists, the two with implanted testicles became aggressive fighting crowing roosters again. This led him to believe hormones were transferred in the blood.

Noting these experiments, French physiologist Charles Edouard Brown-Sequard mashed up the sex glands of dogs and guinea pigs, brewed them in a salt solution, and self-injected them. He died in 1894 a discredited scientist, after claiming these injections gave him a youthful energy which, however, quickly faded. In 1926,

Professor Fred Koch at the University of Chicago experimented with the fractionating, extracting and distilling of hundreds of pounds of bull testicles, where those before him had worked in ounces. In 1935 the Yugoslavian chemist, Leopold Ruzicka, developed the first synthetic testosterone.

It was believed the Germans gave testosterone to their troops to ensure their aggressiveness on the battle field, and ironically these same medications were given to World War II concentration camp victims to help correct starvation and severe negative nitrogen balance.

Anabolic steroids came on the sporting scene in the 1950s, the Eastern Bloc countries being the first noted to experiment in international competition. In the 1952 Summer Olympic Games held in Helsinki, the Soviet Union, appearing in their first Olympic Games and still recovering from the recent world war, surprisingly won three gold medals, three silver, and one bronze in weight-lifting.

American weight-lifting team physician, Dr John Ziegler, noted this at another world weight-lifting championship in Vienna, and came back to the US determined to give American athletes the same chemical combat tools. He worked with a pharmaceutical company to develop Dianabol (methandrostenolone), and began experiments by administering it to America's top weight-lifters at the York Barbell Club in Pennsylvania. Seeing the dangerous side-effects of the drug, he tried to stop this practice, but it was too late. Anabolic steroids had been introduced to the sports world.

Regretfully, it appears that societies have relaxed their condemnation of drug use, and certain substances have become acceptable in social circumstances. Despite governmental controls, these substances now find their way around the world because of the massive profits which can be accrued.

Today, many athletes find themselves under such pressure that they and their coaches (and even their physicians) are tempted to use drugs to stimulate or sedate, to increase or decrease weight, and to help combat the fatigue of a strenuous training program. The rewards of athletic success have become enormous. To the traditional prestige of championship success, we can now add financial benefits accrued in an athletic fund for sporting retirement.

In order to reach the top in both national and international competition, much is demanded from an athlete. A minimum training program requiring a commitment of several hours a day is necessary. In other words, it is hard both physically and mentally. Some athletes cannot handle the pressure and expectations in the chase for medals, places and top results. In the hope of becoming a little better than the other competitors, some athletes, unfortunately, are tempted to use banned doping substances. They begin to use different drugs without reflecting on the risks they are taking. The only sure way to get results is through dedicated exercise training and ingesting proper nutritional fuels. It has been noted that with proper nutrition, the use of proteins and amino acids, as well as supplemental vitamins and minerals, in combination with heavy resistance training, an athlete can over an extended period of time enhance their performance in ways similar to those induced by drugs such as anabolic steroids—but without the adverse side-effects. The drug-free athlete's longevity for competition will also be much greater than that of the doping athlete, who tends to 'burn out' more quickly.

The ultimate responsibility in such matters lies with the athlete. However, supervisors can play a significant role in shaping moral attitudes and values by watching for signs of drug use. The supervisor can be a teacher, coach, team physician, club leader/official or an older athlete. The adult supervisor is a role model and should exercise care in the area of drugs. At all times, behaviour must be exemplary. The supervisor has a responsibility not only for the young person, but also for the institution which the athlete represents.

There are two basic classes of sports drugs. One is restorative drugs, which aid the recovery to the previous state of health and performance. They may enable the athlete to compete despite being injured. Some examples of drugs in this class are pain killers such as aspirin, morphine, muscle relaxants, topical anaesthetics, and anti-inflammatories.

The other class of sports drugs are ergogenic substances. These are additive, and in some cases enable performance to go beyond what would normally be possible. They may be pharmacologic, physiologic, or nutritional. Examples of such substances are anabolic steroids, amphetamines, cocaine, caffeine, and blood doping.

Doping in sport is the deliberate administration of a non-food substance or substances with the purpose of artificially enhancing an athlete's physical and/or mental condition. It can also be the clinical manipulation of natural substances in an athlete's body for the same purpose of falsely enhancing the physical and/or mental condition.

Knowledge of the effects and side-effects of drugs is based mainly on their use in the treatment of different diseases and illnesses. Drugs can never be said to be completely safe. Certain drugs can have such damaging effects on the body's various organs that their use must be limited to very severe disease states. In the treatment of ill people, a drug's positive effects must therefore be weighed against its damaging effects. The selection of a drug by a physician is based on the knowledge that exists regarding different doses, and/or of a different drug's effects and side-effects at certain controlled doses.

Taking a drug in completely different doses, and/or for a different purpose than was intended, increases the risk that the drug will have unwanted side-effects. This applies to a great extent to the drugs that are used for doping. It is therefore vital to be aware of the latest information on the properties of a drug.

What follows is a discussion of the medical uses, effects and side-effects of stimulants, anabolic steroids, and human growth hormone (HGH)—all of which are on the current IOC list of banned substances.

Psychomotor stimulants: amphetamines, cocaine and related substances

Psychomotor stimulants have been used as ergogenics for many years. The first were of plant origin, such as the leaves of the coca plant and the African plant *Catho edulis*. These contain the psychomotor stimulant drugs cocaine and norisoephedrine. Cocaine, a natural derivative of the leaf of the *Erythroxylum coca* plant, was used in ancient rituals by the Incas.

Cocaine is taken in a number of fashions:

• Smoking. A less pure form of cocaine (coca paste) gives a rapid onset 'high' of short duration. To smoke *free-base*, the extract of cocaine is prepared with the use of a volatile solvent such as ether.

• Sniffing. The white powder crystals are inhaled through the nose via a straw or a rolled up piece of paper. The drug is rapidly absorbed through the nasal mucosa for a rapid euphoria. With repeated nasal ingestion, the mucosa are severely damaged in regular users.

• Intravenous. The high peaks out in three to five minutes and the user is vulnerable to risks of intravenous drug abuse such as AIDS and hepatitis (i.e. all 3 forms, Hepatitis B_1, Hepatitis A_1, and Non-A Non-B).

• Crack. This is a very pure form of cocaine that can be smoked or mixed with tobacco, and is very addictive.

Amphetamine (2-phenylisopropylamine) is very similar to naturally occurring stimulants. It was first synthesised in 1887 as a crystalline, white odourless powder. Its derivative, N-methamphetamine, was first produced in 1919. Both of these drugs were used extensively by troops during World War II to fend off fatigue. Some common amphetamines are benzedrine and dexedrine. None of these substances is accepted for sports use. They are classed as stimulants because of the euphoria they cause, which can lead to addiction. The medical uses of these substances are limited to some very uncommon diseases such as depressive insomnia. Central nervous stimulants have, in the past, been used as appetite suppressants, but their effects are short lived and of doubtful value.

Amphetamines, cocaine and related substances increase wakefulness, and suppress feelings of tiredness, through stimulation of the central nervous system (the brain). Users frequently feel exhausted, especially after prolonged periods of use, but in some cases there is agitation and irritability instead. Among misusers, tolerance is quickly built up (the dosage must be steadily increased to produce the same effects). With this there is an increased risk of dangerous changes in mental state, including psychotic reactions. This can manifest as delusions which are often combined with hallucinations.

There is evidence that amphetamines extend aerobic endurance and quicken recovery from fatigue. Hence their use in athletic events which require protracted exertion. However, after the body's warning signals for exhaustion are suppressed there is a high risk of overwork resulting in collapse, and in the worst cases, death. With high concentrations of the drug, endurance capacity can drop to a quasiparalytic state (neuromuscular blockade) culminating in death. Cocaine has many similarities to amphetamines and is highly addictive.

Side-effects

These drugs share relatively common side-effects. These include:

- Addiction
- Restlessness, irritability, dizziness, difficulty in sleeping
- Tiredness and depression when the effects of the drug wear off
- Heart palpitations, profuse sweating
- Dry mouth
- Difficulty with urination
- Rise in blood pressure
- Mydriasis
- Increase in blood sugar
- Increased muscle tone

- Shorter blood coagulation time
- Stimulation of adrenal glands
- Overdose can lead to circulatory collapse, convulsions and death.

Androgenic anabolic steroids

Androgenic anabolic steroids are male hormones. ('Androgenic' meaning to promote masculine characteristics, 'anabolic' referring to promotion of tissue growth.) Hormones have many functions in the body. They can:

- Inactivate or activate enzyme systems
- Change the rates of reactions
- Alter the permeability of cell membranes to certain substances
- Increase or decrease specific enzyme systems
- Influence the genetic material itself.

Research by Dobriner, Rhodes and colleagues in 1974 noted that there were five causal relationships between exogenously administered steroid hormones and cancer. These were:

- They may provide growth of tissue upon which other mechanisms act
- They act in conjunction with other agents as co-factors or promoters
- They may cause tissues themselves to produce carcinogens (cancer cells)
- They may initiate neoplastic change
- They may give rise to neoplasia-inciting metabolites.

Testosterone is the primary male hormone. It has the following effects on males under normal circumstances when produced in the body:

- Associated with the mental disposition of libido, sexual desire, and aggressiveness
- Stimulates growth of target organs
- Promotes protein anabolism
- Determines sexual characteristics: at puberty—larynx enlargement, vocal cord thickening, increase in body hair, increase in muscle mass, increase in oil gland secretion by skin
- Reduces protein catabolism (breakdown, degradation)
- Stimulates spermatogenesis
- Has metabolic effects on muscle, skin, and bone

- Influences closure of epiphyses in long bones
- Increases size of seminiferous tubules and testes
- Aids in development and maintenance of accessory sex organs, including secretory functions, and increase in external genitalia and tubule structures. With decreased androgen, these structures begin to atrophy.
- Causes marked changes in psychological outlook and perspectives, specifically in relation to body image and personal identity.

Testosterone is medically administered when a person's own production of the hormone is abnormally low. It is also used in the treatment of breast cancer in women. In very high doses, testosterone can have a favourable effect on certain life threatening blood disorders.

Testosterone has an anabolic effect. When administered exogenously, this effect is more marked in boys before puberty and in women, than in grown men, because boys and women have very low levels of testosterone in their bodies. Testosterone production within the body is part of a complex hormone regulatory system. When this system operates in a normal way, the individual will have very limited use, if any, for additional testosterone.

Testosterone has a more virilising effect than synthetic anabolic steroids, which among other things, is a disadvantage in medical treatment of women.

Synthetic Anabolic Steroids

Synthetic anabolic steroids are chemical products which are synthesised to have less virilising effects than testosterone, while retaining their anabolic effects. Since anabolic steroids are felt to increase muscular size, strength and power, they are commonly employed in sporting activities requiring these elements. However, due to widespread public exposure, they have found their way into the majority of sporting activities, and their use is relatively common even among those who do not actively participate in sport, but use them for cosmetic reasons—to look better. This, coupled with the *younger* pre-pubescent athlete using this banned substance, leads to some serious potential health risks.

Protein anabolism involves a reduction in the excretion of urea (by-product of protein), without any change in the excretion of uric acid, ammonia, or nitrogen in the faeces. In addition, the excretion of phosphate, calcium, sodium, chloride and potassium is also reduced. However, the anabolic effect does not continue, as the body nitrogen balance eventually returns to normal. At that time a 'wearing off' phase occurs.

When anabolic steroid administration is halted, a 'rebound effect' may occur, with negative nitrogen balance and significant weight loss. The degree to which these conditions occur is a function of dose, medications taken, duration of administration, quantity of drugs ingested, and physiologic state of the subject. There are a variety of different synthetic anabolic androgenic steroid preparations on the market.

Anabolic steroid drugs are taken in a number of ways:

- Stacking—using more than one drug at the same time
- Shotgunning—a hit-or-miss technique
- Tapering—gradually deceasing intake
- Plateauing—term used for the stage when one drug is no longer effective at a certain level
- Blending—mixing of different drugs
- Cycling—for example, going on for a six to eight week period, and then off again for the same time and repeating the cycle.

The build-up of body tissues is stimulated normally by certain endogenous hormones, among others growth hormone and the female and male sex hormones. The effects of synthetic anabolic steroids are similar to the male sex hormone testosterone, but the virilisation effects are less apparent.

The role of anabolic steroids in the strengthening of tissues after a long sickness is still unclear. It is not certain, for example whether a man with normal production of testosterone can utilise increased amounts of exogenous synthetic anabolic substances without decreasing, or stopping altogether, his normal production of male hormones.

The therapeutic uses of anabolic steroids include:

- Surgery. They aid and promote healing, improve appetite, and increase protein synthesis. They also serve as a protective aid for blood-producing bone marrow after malignant tumors have been treated with radiation therapy.
- Skeletal disorders. Anabolic steroids aid and stimulate the formation of protein matrix of the bone; they help to retard the effects of osteoporosis which occurs in the elderly as bone loss.
- Starvation and malnutrition. For individuals who have an insufficient intake of dietary protein. This occurs most in the elderly. Improved appetite results allowing the stimulation of cellular growth. Negative nitrogen balance can be corrected. The patient has an uplifted psychological disposition, and may experience a feeling of well-being.

- Balance therapy. For patients who may have a low hormonal production rate.

Any significant performance-enhancing effects of testosterone or other anabolic steroids in male athletes have not been thus far verified by the few, and considerably incomplete, scientific studies carried out. Scientifically conclusive reports of the effect of anabolic steroids on muscle strength and performance level in women are also lacking. Muscle mass does, however, increase with longterm usage. However, the bulk of steroid ingesting athletes feel steroid drugs can have significant strength and muscle gaining effects.

Anabolic steroid doping has a detrimental effect on many bodily functions including gonadal function, prostate, kidney and liver functions, cardiovascular function, bone growth, and in women, virilising effects can be added to this general list.

Gonadal Function

A reduced sperm production and testicular atrophy occurs soon after anabolic steroid use has started. The amount of this reduction depends on the dose. After the use of anabolic steroids is stopped, as a rule, sperm production does increase again, but very slowly. It is uncertain if the sperm production and fertility ever returns to normal. Sometimes the individual develops a new 'low normal level' of hormone production, and impotence can occur.

Prostate gland

The prostate gland weighs only a few grams at birth, but due to the influence of androgens reaches its full size of about 20 grams by age 20. It remains this size for about 25 years until the fifth decade of life when the second growth spurt occurs. Cancer of the prostate is the second most common malignancy in men over 55 years old, and is the third most common cause of cancer death after carcinomas of the lung and colon.

Although this type of cancer is rare in those under the age of 50, there is evidence to suggest that anabolic steroids may cause a change in the fatal case age distribution, because anabolic steroids cause the prostate to enlarge significantly at a much younger age. Common symptoms of prostate enlargement are dysuria, difficulty in voiding, increased urinary frequency, complete blockage of urinary excretion, back and hip pain, and haematuria.

Kidney disease

Another organ of concern is the kidney, which is important for excretion of wastes as urine. When taking anabolic steroids the body retains significant calcium. There is the possibility of a massive outpouring of calcium when steroid administration ceases, which may contribute to renal calcium stone formation. Warning signs are flank pain and haematuria.

Another disorder known as Wilm's Tumor (nephroblastoma), has been linked with anabolic steroid use. A common kidney tumor in children, it is a very rare and fatal tumor in adults. In half the cases, the condition is diagnosed before the age of 4 (90 per cent before 8). Haematuria, pain, fever, hypertension, and a palpable mass are diagnostic signs of the tumor. Flank, lumbar, or abdominal pain are also early warning signs.

Cardiovascular disease

Heart disease will probably be the most widely noted side-effect with anabolic steroid use. Blood pressure elevates significantly when an individual takes anabolic steroids, due to the retained fluid and increased blood volume. The mechanism for this may be that anabolic drugs may increase blood pressure by a direct inhibition of 11-beta hydroxylation, and consequent overproduction of deoxycorticosterone by the adrenal cortex.

High density lipoproteins (HDL-C) that aid the body in removing cholesterol, and are important to cardiac longevity, are drastically reduced with the use of androgens. A normal level of 45 mg per decilitre commonly falls to as low as 5 in the steroid-ingesting athlete. The low density lipoproteins (LDL-C), as well as cholesterol levels, commonly rise, contributing to increased cardiovascular risk.

This in combination with drugs of a stimulant nature may predispose the athlete to a hazardous cardiovascular incident. In addition, another factor predisposing to atherosclerosis with anabolic steroid use is increased levels of cortisol, possibly by decreased catabolism of cortisol by the liver.

Excess testosterone in the body is converted to oestrogen, and elevated oestrogen levels have been linked to adverse lipoprotein profiles. The change in blood clotting factors that occurs with both male and female sex hormone administration may also have adverse long-term health effects.

Weight-training athletes will hold their breath many times during a lift (valsalva manoeuvre), significantly increasing systemic blood pressure as well as intrathoracic vascular pressure. This may predispose a weakened cardiovascular system with elevated resting blood pressure towards stroke, ruptured aneurysm and haemorrhage.

Liver dysfunction

The liver is the vital detoxifying organ of the body, and where anabolic steroids are broken down, conjugated and metabolised. The liver is responsible for regulation of glucose, storage of glycogen, deamination, transamination, and conversion of nitrogenous wastes to urea so that they can be excreted by the kidneys. In addition, bile is synthesised in the liver, vitamins A, D, E, and K are stored, and there is excretion of bile pigments. The liver is responsible for the destruction of old red blood cells, as well as for a host of other critically important body functions.

Liver damage may occur by two reactions; either as a direct toxic effect (as is the case with anabolic steroids), or from a hypersensitivity reaction. It is felt steroids interfere with the excretory functions of the liver, and this has been documented in both animal and human studies. Some of the major intermediate consequences in anabolic steroid-induced disturbances of excretory function are noted as elevated bilirubin levels, and BSP (bromosulphthalein) retention. Clinically it appears that this is caused primarily by 17-alpha alkylated (oral) steroids.

Serum transaminase levels (SGOT and SGPT, an enzyme closely tied to hepatocellular damage) and alkaline phosphatase are noted to rise with steroid use. If an athlete has a transaminase or alkaline phosphatase level above 150 units/L or a total bilirubin in excess of 2 υmol/L, the steroids should be stopped immediately and clinical follow-up begun.

Oral anabolic steroids have also been implicated in two other serious disorders, peliosis hepatis and liver tumors (hepatocellular carcinoma). With peliosis hepatis, intrahepatic cholestasis develops—the liver cells are unable to excrete conjugated bilirubin and organic anions into the bile ducts, causing bilirubin to accumulate within the liver cells. Some of this is excreted into the liver sinusoids. The liver cells then begin to degenerate, and blood escapes into the spaces forming 'blood pools' or 'blood lakes' in the liver tissue. The liver becomes enlarged and tender. Peliosis is a fatal disorder with death being caused by liver failure.

Hepatocellular carcinoma in steroid-ingesting subjects has been noted. One case was a 26-year-old body builder, another a 37-year-old weight trainer who took anabolic steroids for cosmetic reasons. It appears the steroids do more to promote tumor growth than to initiate neoplasia. However, this is still an area of debate.

The following is a liver dysfunction warning list:

- Look for atrophy or enlargement of lobes of liver
- Change in texture, such as increase in hardness, or nodularity
- Tenderness to palpation
- Tenderness to ballottement (pushing to and fro)
- Jaundice
- Discolouration of the urine; do not confuse with colour change secondary to high vitamin intake
- Abdominal pain of visceral type; pain increased by coughing or movement and usually located in upper right quadrant
- Palmar erythema (red palms), and spider angiomas (brown spider-like blemish on skin) which may reflect acute or chronic liver disease
- Finger clubbing (swelling of flesh at base of nail bed on the fingers)
- Change in mental state or neurologic function.

Gynaecomastia

The large amount of testosterone secondary to exogenous administration of anabolic steroids is converted into the female hormone oestrogen. In the male, this leads to the formation of female breast tissue known as gynaecomastia. This female breast bud may resolve with time following cessation of steroid ingestion, but in some cases requires surgery to remove.

Bone growth

In growing people, that is those under age 20, anabolic steroids can cause premature epiphysial closure at an early stage of growth. Normally, at these early stages, the long bones have a large cartilage portion where certain enzymes are secreted into the immediate intracellular environment to cause mineral deposition and thus calcification. But the epiphyses at the ends of the long bone remain cartilage and continue to divide to make the bone grow longer. Eventually bone replacement will catch up with the cartilage ends causing epiphysial cartilage to disappear, after which there would be no further increase in bone length. Full bone growth usually continues until the mid-twenties. Due to early closure under the influence of anabolic steroids of the growth plate zones of the long body bones, a young athlete may be abnormally short, and this change will be irreversible. Anabolic steroids are given for medical management only in specific circumstances.

Side-effects in women

In females, the virilisation effects from anabolic steroids can be noticed even after a short time. The side effects manifest themselves in the form of:

* Lowering of the voice to a bass level (vocal cord thickening), which is irreversible
* Increased hair growth on the face and a masculine body hair distribution
* Male pattern baldness
* Menstrual disturbances
* Fertility disturbances
* Decrease in breast size, and altered fat distribution
* Clitoral hypertrophy (enlargement), which is irreversible
* Severe acne. Due to an increase in skin oil gland secretion, this can occur in a short period of time. The distribution is typically on the face, back, shoulders and chest, but may extend to the abdomen and even the arms and legs. If not treated properly, lifelong scarring of the epidermis can occur.

Psychogenic behavioral changes

The psychological side-effects of anabolic steroids can be extreme. The individual may become very aggressive and hostile, even to the point of acts of violence, known as 'steroid rage' or 'roid rage'. Criminal cases have actually presented steroid psychosis as a litigation defense for violent or psychotic behavior. The emotional rollercoaster effect is classically exhibited in males. It is common for individuals to suffer from 'reverse anorexia'. This is where no matter what physical stature the athlete achieves (large body weight and size), they still view themselves as small and weak.

Even more devastating is the severe depression that occurs when steroid administration is ceased. Suicidal ideation may be attributed to steroid-induced psychotic depression.

Growth hormone

Human growth hormone (HGH), otherwise known as somatotrophin or somatotrophic hormone (STH) is a polypeptide hormone with a molecular weight of 21 500 (composed of 191 amino acids). It is produced by the anterior division of the pituitary gland.

Growth hormone has its primary effect on growth, but it also influences a number of other functions in the body, among them sugar and fat conversion. In pre-adults, HGH stimulates linear growth of the bone. It also stimulates intracellular transport of amino acids, and causes nitrogen retention, which is a supposed marker of protein anabolism (building). The activity of messenger RNA is affected, which increases protein synthesis in specific cells, and stimulates the intracellular breakdown of body fat so that more fat is used for energy, which has a protein sparing effect.

HGH also stimulates the liver to produce somatomedins which are messenger molecules sometimes referred to as growth factors.

Medically, HGH is administered to prevent dwarfism in children and youths who have a deficiency of the hormone. Prior to the genetically manufactured synthetic HGH, the supply of growth hormone was limited to pituitary gland sources. In spite of this earlier shortage of the drug, its use as a doping agent had already been reported.

Too much growth hormone before puberty leads to excess (height can be over 2.10 metres), while 'acromegaly' develops if the doses of growth hormone are too high after puberty.

Acromegaly is beginning to be noted in athletes, with increased coarsening of facial features, increased size of the nose, lips, tongue and soft facial tissues. An underbite is noted, with enlargement of the mandible and jaw. The forehead becomes more prominent as the orbital ridges and frontal sinuses enlarge, and the fingers and toes widen into a spade-like shape. There is an increase in sweating and sebaceous gland activity, along with small patches of increased skin pigmentation, known as fibromata mollusca.

The growth of the cartilage and soft tissues causes the joint spaces to widen, leading to significant joint pain, along with distortion of body structures, leading to disfigurement.

Organomegaly and visceromegaly (increase in size of organs and viscera) may lead to congestive heart failure. Likewise, there is a risk of diabetes and other metabolic disorders.

It is important to athletes to be aware that much black-market HGH is not in fact, HGH. On numerous occasions, injectable steroids have been substituted for HGH leading to positive doping tests. In some cases, animal HGH (bovine, Rhesus monkey etc.) has been injected. Non-primate HGH is incompatible with the human species. Impure compounds passed off as HGH have caused other serious diseases.

Conclusion

Physicians play a key role in the education of athletes and it is critical that medical personnel should themselves have a thorough understanding of the effects of ergogenics if they are to assist athletes in making informed decisions on their use. Each physician should establish a personal policy on sports drug use, and make it clear to patients.

Those tempted to use drugs to enhance sports performance, or assist in the administration of such drugs to others, can be coerced into correct behavior by the threat of legal actions, doping control at more competitions, and by an increase in the minimum period of ineligibility for the offending athlete. The continuing spread of random testing during training periods is a development to be applauded and encouraged.

If we continue, however, to pursue the problem only through ever-increasing use of doping control, we merely extend the pharmaceutical war. Our laboratories will continue to chase the lead of those prepared to indulge in dangerous 'experimentation'. It is crucial that the problem is traced back to its source and eradicated. Physicians have an important role to play in the fight to rid sport of the life-threatening hazards of drug misuse.

Acknowledgments

Data in this chapter were made possible by the fine past work of scientists who authored:

• The position statements on drugs for the International Federation of Body Builders, the American College of Sports Medicine, and for the National Strength and Conditioning Association of America.

• An anti-doping paper 'Aerling Kamp', by the Swedish Sports Confederation, in cooperation with the Swedish Pharmacy Association. English translation provided by Mr William Glad.

• 'The Control of Drug Abuse in Sport', Drug Control and Teaching Centre, Kings College, University of London—Associate Director, Dr David Cowan.

I would also like to acknowledge sources in the International Olympic Committee, National Academy of Sports Medicine, the International Amateur Athletic Federation, and the International Athletic Foundation.

Finally, I acknowledge my colleague, Professor Manfred Donike, Chairman of the International Olympic Committee's Doping Committee, who provided important data and guidance.

11 Conclusions and recommendations
Saxon White and Ronald Laura

Contemporary theme song from an ABC children's video:
'Roger Ramjet he's our hero
Hero of our nation—'
— provided he takes his routine, Proton energy pill! (Eds)

In Australia, despite the Australian Sports Medicine Federation's survey of 1983, no one has yet taken responsibility for designing a comprehensive national survey that might define the multifaceted components of the problem of drug-taking in sport. Consequently, individuals and organisations with honest intent may make uncoordinated and often inappropriate attempts to correct an ill-defined problem! Moreover, if there is no clear public agreement that the use of drugs in sport is a deviation from approved sporting behaviour, how can one justify any corrective act?

The purpose of the International Congress on Drugs in Sport hosted by the Hunter Academy of Sport was to attempt to bring some understanding of the issues to the Australian public and its sporting experts. The Congress format therefore included two public meetings (the outcomes of which are reported in detail[1] in separately published documents) to allow the public to listen, debate, and make statements. How else could the public express their opinion?

What followed was a demonstration of opinion, encouragement and action. Present were the Lord Mayor of Newcastle, John McNaughton, the New South Wales Minister for Sport, Recreation and Racing, Bob Rowland Smith, and the NSW Minister for Health, Peter Collins, who all indicated that they were against

144

drug-taking in sport. Peter Collins also outlined the NSW government's intentions, then on the drawing board, to amend the Poisons Regulations in relation to the possession of an unlawful supply of steroids. (This was reaffirmed in May 1990, following the death of the 23-year-old Sydney bodybuilder, Maurice Ferranti, through steroid abuse, but changes to the regulations have not occurred as yet).

Mr Steve Haynes, of the Australian Sports Drug Agency in Canberra, referred to the statement (made the day before the Congress, 21 August, 1989) by Senator Grahame Richardson that the Commonwealth government had acted on the initial recommendations of Senator Black's Committee of Inquiry into Drugs in Sport concerning the establishment of (i) a uniform Drugs in Sport policy across Australia and (ii) an independent body to educate the sporting and general community on the dangers of performance-enhancing drugs. The government would also urge the independent sampling and testing of sportspeople at all levels for drug usage in sport. This was followed through during the winter of 1990 particularly in relation to testing Rugby League players, with well publicised and controversial sequelae, mainly in relation to the rights of the players where confidentiality and the media were concerned. The drug budget for the Anti-Drugs Campaign had, in 1989, been raised to $4 million for the ensuing four years. Steve Haynes and his team then outlined the educational processes being initiated, and spoke on the drug data underpinning these processes.

Senator Black's announcement that a national survey would be carried out to define the details of the problem at large was met with general acclaim. The wisdom of such a measure was obvious by halfway through the Congress, by which time it was clear that the public in Australia, and probably internationally, had no real base of information of the controversial, multifaceted issues complicating policy decisions concerning drugs in sport. And this was the likely reason underlying the lack of a consistent, positive Australian, international, and IOC policy, in which rules, guidelines (for athletes, coaches and the general community, including physicians advising athletes), and testing procedures with penalties might achieve some credibility.

Congress delegates spent four days in exhaustive discussions of possible solutions to the problems raised. It was agreed in our most pessimistic but lucid moments over coffee, that the driven mind of some modern athletes recognised no conventions, no guidelines, or laws. But on the other hand, if the IOC could take the positive anti-drug stance of many modern Olympians (as typified by Sebastian Coe's statement at Seoul), and network a positive philosophy and guidance internationally (e.g. with the Australian Olympic Federation), there was hope. What now follows are the formal recommendations that were arrived at by six interactive groups seeking solutions to the final problems as they emerged due to Congress debate. These final problems were identified by the Congress Organising Committee who placed them on notice boards in the coffee venue, with the request that delegates choose their topic and enrol as group participants. The final recommendations were presented later to the Congress delegates by the group rappoteur in a Plenary Session for comment, refinement, acceptance and priority listing.

Recommendation 1

That the International Olympic Committee (IOC) provide a coherent philosophical framework within which the IOC position on doping can be justified and consistently applied.

The philosophy should embrace educational programs, drug-testing and penalties. The determination of such a philosophy might require the creation of a specific advisory body incorporating philosophers, scientists of various persuasions, and above all, contemporary champion athletes to consider concepts of 'fair play' and 'unfair advantage' as it relates to competition at the highest human level. It is perceived that an appropriate philosophical framework would take into account ethical issues concerned with, for example, genetic engineering, as well as the problems of performance-boosting aids including drugs.

The advisory body should also consider effective international communications and decision-making processes and ensure consistency of recommendations and value systems.

Recommendation 2

1 *That a national survey concerning drug-taking in sport be undertaken as a matter of urgency.*

The last survey was undertaken by the Australian Sports Medicine Federation in 1983. While the results were most useful, several criticisms levelled at this survey were found to be valid. The above recommendation incorporates the notion that:

• the coming survey should be designed by leading Australian professionals in the field of behavioural science
• the survey should be coordinated with the participation of

organisations relevant to target groups e.g. Department of Education in relation to school children, and national sporting organisations in relation to athletes

- educational programs would be developed using the data from such surveys
- drug testing programs would be developed using data from the survey
- the results of the survey would be used to develop policy with respect to alternative strategies for detecting drug-taking, given that the responses to the survey can be open to bias
- the results of the survey would be used to formulate follow-up surveys and strategies to monitor the effectiveness of the educational and other programs put in motion by the original survey data.

2 *That the IOC be consulted in coordinating State, or Commonwealth, initiatives with IOC policy concerning modification of drug-taking behaviour.*

3 *That the IOC be encouraged to bring the heads of accredited drug-testing laboratories together for consultation regarding policy formulation.*

Such officials should participate in:

- determining the philosophy of *prevention* of drug-taking in sport
- sharing information concerning advances in new substances purported to be performance-boosting aids
- sharing information concerning advances in detection processes.

Recommendation 3

That in the case of children, the primary goal should aim at prevention through education.

This recommendation incorporates education in the first instance of sporting organisations and in particular, their administrators and coaches. In the second instance, the children themselves should be targeted by educational strategies brought to bear through schools, and through community sporting organisations (clubs, commercial sporting organisations, State departments of sport and recreation etc.)

The educational strategies should include the school curricula and the assessment of these curricula, and incorporate learning about:

- personal development (attitudes and behaviour in sport)
- supposed performance-boosting aids themselves, their risks to health, their possible advantages (e.g. in the case of diet), and alternative performance-boosting strategies
- the philosophy of sport in relation to fair play, winning and losing, how to compete, the history of Australian and international sport, and the philosophy of the IOC and national and international sporting networks
- the role of information networks such as newspapers, magazines, radio and television as communication processes
- the use of role models for determining behaviour.

Recommendation 4

1 *That the principle be followed of avoiding unnecessary government regulation/control.*

2 *That strategies for self-regulation should be the key approach to the problem.*

3 *That sporting organisations should include an appeal mechanism in the articles of association.*

At least in Australia, a systematic approach to defining guidelines should be initiated:

- This could be a Commonwealth initiative but would require before commencing agreed participation of athletes, sports leaders (coaches, referees etc. and administrators), health, medical and law professionals, and finally, of government. This may involve strategic and specially programmed conferences with clear goals and processes to ensure useful outcomes
- Recommendations would necessarily involve policy agreed between states and at the national level, and in keeping with IOC policy (and thereby with the policies of other countries)
- The implementation of the agreed policy would need to be share-funded by State and Commonwealth governments, on the grounds that as in health funding, the implementation of policy with respect to performance-boosting aids in sport affects all citizens at all ages and of both sexes, i.e. it is a national, community issue
- Where appropriate the policy should become law, and be implemented through states, regions and local i.e. sports councils
- Note was made of the failure of the present guidelines and regulations to control the use of performance-boosting aids
- It was considered that self-regulation was the best method of

controlling the abuse of performance-boosting aids, and acknowledged that the success of such an approach could only follow after a major health education approach within the sporting community, and indeed the wider community of Australia

• Therefore, the guidelines and regulations of the future should continue to support in principle the protection of the athlete, and in this regard, an appeal mechanism should be introduced into the system if this is not present already. Individual sports for example should recommend changes to their articles of association for this purpose.

Recommendation 5

1 *That athletes in training be subjected to 'out-of-competition', unannounced testing.*

2 *That the acquisitions of body tissue (fluid etc.) samples be tied securely to the identity of athletes.*

Such security should be established by:

• an international central register of athletes

• a face photograph, name and number for each athlete

• an additional face photograph at the time of the test.

3 *That athletes be subjected to uniform rules concerning training and competition.*

This would be a process in which

• the IOC plays a visible, policy implementing role

• the role of the IOC is supported by National governments (and their associated State or Territory etc governments, and where appropriate, local governments)

• the implementation of IOC policy involves a public relations arm specifically to place the rules of competition, training and penalties in relation to performance-boosting aids in a philosophical perspective within the framework of Olympic ideals.

4 *That the IOC seek the cooperation of member nations to provide funds for the implementation of Recommendations 1, 2 and 3.*

Recommendation 6

1 *That a consistent policy be formulated regarding research into performance-boosting aids, incorporating the new ethics of drug-taking in sport and the information concerning known relationships between drugs and performance-enhancement.*

This should be a prerequisite before specific research into pharmaco-physiology is mounted.

2 *That research should be contract and applied using multidisciplinary teams.*

It was seen that traditional approaches to research of performance-boosting by drugs would do little in providing long-term solutions to the problem. Nevertheless, to the extent that knowledge concerning the effects of these drugs is essential for policy development and the formulation of accurate educational programs, contract, target research was essential. Multidisciplinary teams of behavioural scientists, pharmacologists, physiologists and biochemists were essential. Flexibility and speed was necessary to keep pace with new developments.

Appendix A—First national congress on socioethical and medical aspects of drugs in sport—Congress program

Tuesday, 22 August 1989: QUEENS WHARF CONVENTION
CENTRE, NEWCASTLE

AM

9.00   Registration: Morning Tea

10.45   Opening comments and meeting structure
PERFORMANCE AIDS: INTERNAL AND
EXTERNAL INFLUENCES
—Professor Saxon White

1.15   *Keynote Address:* THE FUTURE OF THE OLYMPIC
MOVEMENT
—Professor Arnold Beckett

PM

12.15   Discussion

12.30   Lunch: Elizabeth's Restaurant

1.30   OFFICIAL OPENING OF CONGRESS in presence of
Alderman John McNaughton
Chair: Professor Saxon White

Mr George Keegan, M.P.
The Hon. Peter Collins, M.P.
The Hon. Bob Rowland Smith, M.P.

2.00   *Plenary Session:* THE SCOPE AND LIMITS OF THE
        DRUG PROBLEM IN SPORT
        Panel: Senator John Black, Dr Brian Corrigan and
        Mr Steve Haynes

3.30   Discussion

3.45   Afternoon Tea

4.15   *Keynote Address:* PSYCHOLOGICAL ASPECTS OF
        DRUGS IN SPORT
        —Dr L Scott Frazier
        Chair: Professor Ronald Laura

5.15   Discussion

5.30   MEET THE MEDIA

6.00   Informal Dinner

7.30   *Public Forum*: THE DRUG-SPORT CONNECTION:
        SHOULD WE BE PLUGGED IN?
        Panel: Dr Ken Donald, Ms Dawn Fraser,
        Dr L Scott Frazier, Professor Vernon Howard,
        Mr Craig Johnston, Mrs Robyn Leggatt,
        Mr Mark Richards, Mr Alex Watson,
        Mr John Knipe, Mayor Ivan Welsh, Mr Henry
        Meskauskas
        Chair: Mr Norman May

Wednesday, 23 August 1989: DAVID MADDISON CLINICAL
                             SCIENCES BUILDING,
                             NEWCASTLE

AM

8.30   Mount Posters: Theme: Drugs, Performance,
        mechanisms of action

9.00   *Keynote Address:* WHAT ARE THE DRUGS, BEING
        USED, HOW DO THEY WORK AND WHAT DO

THEY DO?
—Dr David Cowan
Chair: Dr Brian Corrigan

10.00 Discussion

10.30 Morning Tea: Posters

11.00 THEME: DRUGS, PERFORMANCE, MECHANISMS
OF ACTION
Free Papers—Dr Dick Telford,
Dr Tony Quail, Dr David Cowan, and Professor Saxon
White
Chair: Dr Ken Donald

PM

12.30 Lunch: Posters
Personal nomination for workshop groups, by topic

2.00 *Panel Debate:* THE CASE FOR AND AGAINST
DOPING IN SPORT
Dr Brian Corrigan, Dr Ken Donald, Dr Tony Millar,
Mr Wayne Pearce, Dr Brian Sando, Mr Jack Newton
and Mr Alex Watson
Chair: Dr Robert Goldman

3.00 Discussion

3.30 Afternoon Tea

4.00 *Workshops* (concurrent): Small groups identify and
refine specific problems of Drugs in Sport

5.00 *Post Workshop Plenary Session:* Documentation of
Problems
Group Secretaries Report
Chair: Professor Ronald Laura

8.00 *Hypothetical:*
DRUGS IN SPORT—THE BIRTH OF SUPERMAN
Panel: Professor Arnold Beckett, Mr Ken Cole,
Dr Brian Corrigan, Dr David Cowan, Dr Ken Donald,
Dr L Scott Frazier, Dr Philip Furey,
Professor Vernon Howard, Mr Craig Johnston,
Dr Tony Millar, Mr Jack Newton, Mr Wayne Pearce,

Dr Brian Sando, Mr Alex Watson, Miss Elizabeth
Toohey
Chair: Professor Ronald Laura

Thursday, 24 August 1989: DAVID MADDISON CLINICAL
SCIENCES BUILDING,
NEWCASTLE

AM

9.00   *Keynote Address:* THE ADVERSE EFFECTS OF
PERFORMANCE BOOSTING DRUGS ON THE
HUMAN SYSTEM
—Dr Robert Goldman

10.00   Discussion
Chair: Dr David Cowan

10.15   Morning Tea: Posters

10.45   *Keynote Address:* ETHICAL ISSUES OF DRUGS IN
SPORT
—Professor Vernon Howard
Chair: Dr L Scott Frazier

11.45   Discussion

PM

12.00   Lunch: Posters

1.00   TEACHING HOSPITAL GRAND ROUNDS: OPEN
FORUM
Case Studies: Dr Tony Millar and Dr Phillip Furey
Howard

2.15   *Keynote Address:* IS THERE A PLACE FOR DRUGS
IN THE PERFORMING ARTS?
—Miss Maina Gielgud (Video Address)
—Miss Elizabeth Toohey
Chair: Professor Saxon White

2.45   Discussion

3.30   Afternoon Tea

4.00   *Keynote Address*: THE RIGHTS OF MEN AND
          WOMEN
          —Mr Lloyd Waddy
          Chair: Mrs Robyn Leggatt

4.30   Discussion
          Posters taken down

5.00   MEET THE MEDIA

7.30   CONGRESS DINNER: THE NEWCASTLE CLUB
          Address: The Hon Bob Rowland Smith, M.P.
          Reply on behalf of the 'Athletes': Mr Lloyd Waddy,
          Q.C.
          Chair: Mr Ken Brown

Friday, 25 August 1989: DAVID MADDISON CLINICAL
                          SCIENCES BUILDING, NEWCASTLE

AM

9.30   *Keynote Address:* TOWARDS A NEW PHILOSOPHY
          OF SPORT
          —Professor Ronald Laura
          Chair: Professor Vernon Howard

10.30   Discussion

11.00   Morning Tea

11.30   *Plenary Panel*: WHAT SHOULD BE DONE?
          Professor Arnold Beckett, Dr David Cowan, Dr L
          Scott Frazier, Dr Bob Goldman, Professor Vernon
          Howard, Mr Craig Johnston, Dr Brian Sando and Mr
          Alex Watson
          Chair: Dr Brian Corrigan

PM

1.00   Lunch:

2.00   Workshops: SOLUTIONS

3.00   Plenary Sessions from Workshops (feedback)

4.00   Afternoon Tea

4.30   CONGRESS ROUND UP AND CONCLUDING
        COMMENTS
        Led by Professor Saxon White

4.45   CLOSURE OF MEETING: Mr George Souris, M.P.

Appendix B—Satellite program

**THE HUNTER POSTGRADUATE MEDICAL INSTITUTE
'DRUG ABUSE IN HUNTER SPORT'**

Saturday, 26 August 1989: DAVID MADDISON CLINICAL
SCIENCES BUILDING CASE
STUDY THEATRE

PM

1.30   Registration

1.50   Introduction and Welcome
        Chairman: Professor Saxon White

2.00   DRUG ABUSE AFFECTING CHILDREN IN SPORT
        THE U.S.A. EXPERIENCE
        —Dr Robert Goldman

2.40   EXPERIENCE AT LEWISHAM INSTITUTE OF
        SPORT—INTERFACE WITH DRUG ABUSE
        —Dr Tony Millar

3.00   DRUG ABUSE IN AUSTRALIAN OLYMPIC
        ATHLETES
        —Dr Brian Corrigan

3.30   Afternoon Tea

4.00   Group discussion of problems

5.00   Conclusion: Professor Saxon White

         COCKTAIL HOUR: Meet the Speakers
         Informal get-together: meet and talk with guests over a
         little wine and cheese.

References

Chapter 1

1. Hanley D.F. (1979) The History of the Olympic Games, in *Sports Medicine and Physiology*, ed RH Strauss, Philadelphia: WB Saunders p. 396.
2. ibid.
3. Harris H.A. (1979) *Greek Athletes and Athletics*, Westport: Greenwood pp 180–81.
4. Axthelm P (1988) Using Chemistry to Get the Gold, *Newsweek*, 26th July, pp 88–89.
5. Beckett A.H. (1983) Sports Injuries: Drugs in Sport, *British Journal of Hospital Medicine*, 29(3), p. 221.
6. ibid.
7. Corrigan B. (1988) *Drugs in Sport*, Balgowlah, NSW: The Medicine Group, p. 3.
8. Beckett op. cit.
9. Beckett op. cit.
10. Goldman B. (1988) *The E Factor*, New York: William Morrow, pp. 31–32, 103.
11. Chelminski R. (1988) The Shocking Stain on Internation Athletics, *Readers' Digest*, September, pp. 132–134.
12. Murray T.H. (1983) The Coercive Power of Drugs in Sport, *Hastings Center Report*, August, p. 25
13. ibid.
14. ibid.
15. Axthelm op. cit.
16. Chelminski op. cit.
17. Axthelm op. cit.

18. Courson S. (1984) The Death of Sport, *Sports Illustrated*, May 11 p. 52.
19. Chelminski op. cit.
20. Attwood A. (1988) Doped or Duped, *Time*, October 3, p. 52.
21. Chelminski op. cit.
22. Chelminski op. cit.
23. *Anabolic Steroids in Australian Sport*, 1987 SAA Research (Pamphlet in which authors, place of publication, etc. are deliberately omitted)
24. Chelminski op. cit.
25. Chaikin T. with Telender R. (1988) *The Nightmare of Steroids, Sports Illustrated*, November, 19, p. 86.
26. Telander R. and Noden M. (1989) The Death of An Athlete, *Sports Illustrated*, February 20, p. 14.
27. Murray op. cit.
28. Attwood op. cit.
29. Goldman B. (1988) Steroids in Sports, *USA Today*, December 16, p. 32.
30. Goldman op. cit.
31. Deming A. (1988) Wonderful World of Drugs, *Bulletin*, September 20, p. 105.

Chapter 3

1. All tables and figures in this chapter derived from documents and proceedings of IOC Medical Commission.

Chapter 6

1. Coyle E.F. (1984) Ergogenic aids. *Clinics in Sports Medicine*, 3: 731–742.
2. Kuchenski R. (1983) Biochemical actions of amphetamine and other stimulants, in Creese I. (ed): *Stimulants: Neurochemical, Behavioral, and Clinical Perspectives*, New York: Raven Press, pp 31–61.
3. Smith G.M., Beecher U.K. (1959) Amphetamine sulfate and athletic performance. 1. Objective effects. *JAMA* 170: 542–557.
4. Williams M.H. (1974) *Drugs and Athletic Performance*, Springfield, Il, Charles C. Thomas.
5. Chandler J.V. & Blair S.N. (1980) The effects of amphetamines on selected physiological components related to athletic success. *Medicine and Science in Sports and Exercise* 12: 65–69.
6. Bhagat B., Wheeler N. (1973) Effect of amphetamine on the swimming endurance of rats. *Neuropharmacology* 12: 711–713.
7. Gerald M.C. (1978) Effects of (+)-amphetamine on the treadmill endurance performance of rats. *Neuropharmacology* 17: 703–704.
8. Bravo E.L. (1988) Phenylpropanolamine and other over-the-counter vasoactive compounds. *Hypertension* 11(3) Suppl II: 7–10.
9. Pentel P.R., Asinger R.W., Benowitz N.L. (1985) Propranolol antagonism of phenylpropanolamine-induced hypertension. *Clinical Pharmacology and Therapeutics* 37: 488–494.

10. Lopes J.M., Aubier M., Jardim J., Aranda J.V., Macklem P.T. (1983) Effect of caffeine on skeletal muscle function before and after fatigue. *Journal of Applied Physiology: Respiratory, Environmental and Exercise Physiology* 54(5): 1303-1305.
11. Wood D.S. (1978) Human skeletal muscle: Analysis of Ca^{2+} regulation in skinned fibers using caffeine. *Experimental Neurology* 58: 218-230.
12. Goldstein A., Warren R., Kaizer S. (1965) Psychotropic effects of caffeine in man. I. Individual differences in sensitivity to caffeine-induced wakefulness. *Journal of Pharmacology and Experimental Therapeutics* 149: 156-159.
13. Costill D.K., Dalsky G.P., Fink W.J. (1978) Effects of caffeine ingestion on metabolism and exercise performance. *Medicine and Science in Sports* 10: 155-158.
14. Ivy J.L., Costill D.L., Fink W.J., et al (1979) Influence of caffeine and carbohydrate feedings on endurance performance. *Medicine and Science in Sports* 11: 6-11.
15. O'Neill F.T., Hynak-Hankinson M.T., Gorman T. (1986) Research and application of current topics in sports nutrition. *Journal of the American Dietetic Association* 86: 1007-1015.
16. Rall T.W. (1982) Evolution of the mechanism of action of methylxanthines: from calcium mobilizers to antagonists of adenosine receptors. *Pharmacologist* 24: 277-287.
17. Brown R. and Partington J. (1942) A psychometric comparison of narcotic addicts with hospital attendants. *Journal of General Psychology* 27: 71.
18. Appenzeller O., Standefer J., Appenzeller J., et al (1980) Neurology of endurance training. V. Endorphins. *Neurology* (NY) 30: 418-419.
19. Glasser W. (1976) *Positive addiction*, New York: Harper & Row.
20. Kaiser P. (1984) Physical performance and muscle metabolism during β-adrenergic blockade in man. *Acta Physiologica Scandinavica* 536 (Suppl): 1.
21. Haupt H.A., Rovere G.D. (1984) Anabolic steroids: a review of the literature. *American Journal of Sports Medicine* 1 (6): 469-484.
22. Wilson J.D. (1988) Androgen abuse by athletes. *Endocrine Review* 9: 181-199.
23. Ryan A.J. (1976) Athletics. Anabolic-androgenic steroids. ed Kochakian C.D. *Handbook of Experimental Pharmacology*, Springer-Verlag 43: 525-534 and 723-725.
24. Vanhelder W.P., Radomski M.W., Goode R.C. (1984) Growth hormone responses during intermittent weight lifting exercise in men. *European Journal of Applied Physiology and Occupational Physiology* 53: 31-34.
25. Vanhelder W.P., Casey K., Goode R.C. et al (1986). Growth hormone regulation in two types of aerobic exercise of equal oxygen uptake. *European Journal of Applied Physiology and Occupational Physiology* 55: 236-239.
26. Daughaday W.H. (1985) The anterior pituitary, in Wilson J.D., Foster D.W. (eds): *Williams Textbook of Endocrinology*, ed 7. Philadelphia: W.B. Saunders Co, pp 568-613.

27. Hughes J.P., Friesen H.G. (1985) The nature and regulation of the receptors for pituitary growth hormone. *Annual Review of Physiology* 47: 483–499.
28. Wilkes D., Gledhill N., Smyth R. (1983) Effect of acute induced metabolic alkalosis on 800m racing time. *Medicine and Science in Sports and Exercise* 15: 277–280.
29. Reeds P.J., Hay S.M., Dorward P.M., et al (1988) The effect of B-agonists and antagonists on muscle growth and body composition of young rats (Rattus sp.). *Comparative Biochemistry and Physiology* 89C: 337–341.

Chapter 7

1. Ullyot J. (1974) Women's secret weapon: fat. *Runners World* 9: 22–23.
2. Gorski et al (1976) The effect of estradiol on carbohydrate utilisation during prolonged exercise in rats. *Acta Physiologica Polonica.*, 27: 361–367.
3. Gillespie C.A. and Edgerton V.R. (1970) The role of testosterone in exercise-induced glycogen supercompensation. *Hormone and Metabolism Research.* 2: 364–366.
4. Brown W.J. et al (1986) Metabolic patterns in endurance exercise—a role for the sex hormones? In: *Sports Science.* Ed. Watkins J. et al London, New York: E. & F.N. Spon, pp. 23–29.
5. White S.W. (1987) Exercise and the heart in hypertension. In: *The Heart and Hypertension.* Ed. Messerli F.H., New York: Yorke Medical Books, pp. 435–446.
6. Ayers J.W.T. et al (1985) Anthropomorphic, hormonal, and psychologic correlates of semen quality in endurance-trained male athletes. *Fertility and Sterility*, 43: 917–921.
7. Buchanan A. et al (1989) Cardiorespiratory-endocrine correlates of menstrual irregularity in teenage ballet dancers. *Proceedings of the Australian Physiological and Pharmacological Society*, 20: 180P.
8. Jennings G.L. et al (1984) Effects of changes in physical activity on blood pressure and sympathetic tone. *Journal of Hypertension*, 2, Suppl. 3: 139–141.
9. Brown W.J., Gazibarich G.J., Husain R. et al (1988) Effects of participation in a commercial fitness programme on risk factors for cardiovascular disease. 17th ACHPER Conference, Canberra, 1988. Abstracts p. 59 ACHPER, Adelaide.
10. Cann C.E. et al (1984) Decreased spinal mineral content in amenorrheic women. *Journal of the American Medical Association*, 251, 626–629.
11. Shangold M et al (1990) Evaluation and Management of Menstrual Dysfunction in Athletes. *Journal of the American Medical Association.* 263, 1665–1669.

Chapter 8

1. Watson J.D. and Crick F. (1953) Molecular Structure of Nucleic Acids, *Nature*, April 25, pp. 41–48.
2. Danielli J.F. (1971) Artificial Synthesis of New Life Forms, *Bulletin of Atomic Scientists*, December, pp. 21–22.
3. Hood L. (1990) Gene Location and Gel Electrophoresis, *Science News*, March 8, pp. 148–149.
4. ibid.
5. Schutz M.C. (1989) Fat Gene Cloned, *UCLA* Newsletter, August.
6. ibid.
7. Yoxen E. (1988) *The Gene Business*, New York: Oxford Press, pp. 62–63, 89–91, 104–05, 34.
8. ibid.
9. Kevles D.J. (1985) *In the Name of Eugenics*, Los Angeles: University of California, pp. 240–249, 254–258.
10. Yoxen (1988) op. cit.
11. Howard T. and Rifkin J. (1980) *Who Should Play God?*, New York: Dell, pp. 24–28, 111–112, 159, 167–168, 174–176.
12. Rorvik D., 1975 *In His Image*, N.Y. Collins.
13. Howard and Rifkin (1980) op. cit.
14. Yoxen (1988) op. cit.
15. ibid.
16. Halacy Jr. Ds *Genetic Revolution* (1986) New York, Oxford Univ. Press.
17. Yoxen (1958) op. cit.
18. Watson J.D. (1988) *The DNA Story: A Documentary History of Gene Cloning*, New York: Freeman, p. 236–239.
19. ibid.
20. ibid.
21. ibid.
22. ibid.
23. ibid.
24. Singer P. and Wells D. (1984) *The Reproduction Revolution*, Oxford: Oxford Univ Press, p. 84.
25. Howard and Rifkin (1980) op. cit.
26. ibid.
27. ibid.
28. Yoxen (1958) op. cit.
29. Howard and Rifkin (1980) op. cit.
30. ibid.
31. Kevles D.J. (1985) op. cit.
32. Howard and Rifkin (1980) op. cit.
33. Yoxen (1958) op. cit.

Chapter 9

1. Strauss R.H. (ed) (1987) *Drugs and Performance in Sports.* Philadelphia: W.B. Saunders Co.
2. Asken M.J. (1988) Dying to Win: *The Athlete's Guide to Safe and Unsafe Drugs in Sport.* Washington DC: Acropolis Books Ltd.
3. Johnson L.D. O'Malley P.M. & Bachman T.G. (1989) High School Seniors Illicit Drug Use Down. In *APA Monitor* Washington DC: American Psychological Association, p. 33
4. Catlin D.H. (1987) Detection of Drug Use by Athletes. *Drugs and Performance in Sports,* RH Strauss (ed), Philadelphia: WB Saunders Co. pp 103–120
5. Wells S.J. (1984) Caffeine: Implications of Recent Research for Clinical Practice. *American Journal of Orthopsychiatry,* 54: 375–389.
6. American Psychiatric Association (1987) *Diagnostic and Statistical Manual of Mental Disorders,* 3rd ed—revised, Washington, DC.
7. Bussuk E.L. & Schoonover S.C. (1977) *The Practitioners Guide to Psychoactive Drugs.* New York: Plenum Publishing Co.
8. Mandell A.J. (1979) The Sunday Syndrome: A Unique Pattern of Amphetamine Abuse Indigenous to Professional Football. In DE Smith (ed), *Amphetamine Use, Misuse and Abuse,* Boston: G.K. Hall & Co. pp 218–227
9. Bussuk and Schoonover (1977) op. cit.
10. Snyder S.H. (1979) Amphetamine Psychosis: A 'Model Schizophrenia' Mediated by Catecholamines. *Amphetamine Use, Misuse and Abuse,* D.E. Smith (ed), Boston: G.I. Hall & Co. pp 189–204
11. American Psychiatric Association (1987) op. cit.
12. Jones E. (1953) *The Life and Work of Sigmund Freud,* Vol 1, New York: Basic Books.
13. Kornetsky C. (1976) Pharmacology: *Drugs Affecting Behavior,* New York: John Wiley & Sons.
14. Johnson et al. (1989) op. cit.
15. American Psychiatric Association (1987) op. cit.
16. Lombardo T.A. (1987) Depressants. *Drugs & Performance in Sports,* R.H. Strauss (ed), Philadelphia: WB Saunders Co. pp 87–102
17. American Psychiatric Association (1987) op. cit.
18. ibid.
19. Kornetsky (1976) op. cit.
20. Bassuk and Schoonover (1977) op. cit.
21. *Physician's Desk Reference* (1989), 43rd ed, New Jersey; Medical Economics Company.
22. Johnson W.O. & Moore K. (1988). The Loser. *Sports Illustrated,* October 3, pp 21–27.
23. Wilson J.D. & Griffin J.E. (1980) The Use and Misuse of Androgens, *Metabolism,* 29: 1278–1295.
24. Taylor W.N. (1987) Synthetic Anabolic-Androgenic Steroids: A Plea for Controlled Substance Status. *The Physician and Sports Medicine,* 15: (5), 140–148.

25. Buckley W.E., Yesalis C.E., Friedly K.E., Anderson W.A., Streit A.L. & Wright J.E. (1988) Estimated prevalence of anabolic steroid use among male high school seniors. *Journal of American Medical Association,* 260 (23), 3441–3445.
26. Lamb D.R. (1984) Anabolic Steroids in Athletics: How Well do They Work and How Dangerous are They? *American Journal of Sports Medicine,* 12: 83–102.
27. National Collegiate Athletic Association (1985) The Substance Use and Abuse Habits of College Student-Athletes. Washington DC.
28. Chaikin T. & Telander R. (1988) The Nightmare of Steroids. *Sports Illustrated,* October 24, pp 83–102.
29. Olweas D., Mattsson A., Schalling D. & Low H. (1988) Circulating Testosterone Levels and Aggression in Adolescent Males: A Causal Analysis. *Psychosomatic Medicine,* 50: 261–272.
30. Pope H.G. Jr & Katz D.L. (1988) Affective and Psychotic Symptoms Associated with Anabolic Steroid Use. *American Journal of Psychiatry,* 145: 487–490.
31. Lamb (1984) op. cit.
32. Fuller J.R. & LaFountaine M.J. (1987) Performance-Enhancing Drugs in Sport: A Different Form of Drug Abuse. *Adolescence,* 12: 969–976.
33. ibid.

Chapter 10

1. Bartimole J. (1988) Drugs and the Athlete ... A Losing Combination, Mission, Kansas, *National Collegiate Athletic Association,* p. 4.
2. Loverock P. (1989) The Athlete of the Future, *Los Angeles Times Magazine,* 19 March, pp. 12–23, 26–27, 43–46.
3. ibid. p. 23.
4. Kant I. (1987) *Fundamental Principles of the Metaphysic of Morals,* tr T.K. Abott, Buffalo, New York: Prometheus, (first published in 1785.)
5. Lockwood A.H. (1989) Medical Problems of Musicians, *The New England Journal of Medicine,* 26 January , pp. 221–248.
6. Scheffler I. (1985) *Of Human Potential,* London: Routledge & Kegan Paul, pp. 46–51.
7. Johnson W.O. & Moore K. (1988) The Loser, *Sports Illustrated,* 3 October, pp. 22–23.
8. ibid.
9. Howard V.A. (1981) Habits, Risks and Responsibilities: A Philosophical Overview, *Analysis of Consumer Policy,* ed George Berman, Philadelphia: publication of the Wharton School of Business, University of Pennsylvania.
10. Hepburn R.W. (1967) Philosophical Ideas of Nature, *The Encyclopedia of Philosophy,* Vol 5, ed Paul Edwards, New York: Macmillian, pp. 454, 456.
11. ibid.
12. Mill J.S. (1958) *Essays on Nature,* ed with intro by George Naknikian, New York: Liberal Arts Press, first published in 1874.

13. Nagel T. (1979) Sexual Perversion, *Mortal Questions*, Cambridge: Cambridge University Press, p. 50.
14. Wollheim R. (1967) Natural Law, *The Encyclopedia of Philosophy*, Vol 5, ed Paul Edwards, New York: Macmillian.

Chapter 11

1. The Proceedings of the 1st public meeting, "THE DRUG-SPORT CONNECTION: SHOULD WE BE PLUGGED IN?"(chaired by Norman May, international sporting commentator) and the 2nd, "THE BIRTH OF SUPERMAN"(moderated by Professor Ronald Laura) have been published by and may be obtained from The Hunter Academy of Sport, PO Box 2136, DANGAR, NSW 2309, Australia, as separate documents at a small cost [see Prolegomenon]).

INDEX